Healing Our Hormones, Healing Our Lives

Solutions for
Common Hormonal Conditions

D0556273

First published by O Books, 2009
O Books is an imprint of John Hunt Publishing Ltd., The Bothy, Deershot Lodge, Park Lane, Ropley,
Hants, SO24 0BE, UK
office1@o-books.net
www.o-books.net

Distribution in:

UK and Europe
Orca Book Services
orders@orcabookservices.co.uk
Tel: 01202 665432 Fax: 01202 666219
Int. code (44)

USA and Canada
NBN
custserv@nbnbooks.com
Tel: 1 800 462 6420 Fax: 1 800 338 4550

Australia and New Zealand
Brumby Books
sales@brumbybooks.com.au
Tel: 61 3 9761 5535 Fax: 61 3 9761 7095

Far East (offices in Singapore, Thailand,
Hong Kong, Taiwan)
Pansing Distribution Pte Ltd
kemal@pansing.com
Tel: 65 6319 9939 Fax: 65 6462 5761

South Africa
Alternative Books
altbook@peterhyde.co.za
Tel: 021 555 4027 Fax: 021 447 1430

Text copyright Linda Crockett 2008

Design: Stuart Davies
Cover Logo: Kathy Phillips, Sharon, CT

ISBN: 978 1 84694 168 9

A CIP catalogue record for this book is available
from the British Library.

Printed by Digital Book Print

O Books operates a distinctive and ethical publishing philosophy in
all areas of its business, from its global network of authors to
production and worldwide distribution.

Healing Our Hormones, Healing Our Lives

Solutions for
Common Hormonal Conditions

Linda Crockett

BOOKS

Winchester, UK
Washington, USA

CONTENTS

Chapter 3 The Spiritual

Chapter 4 Healing Ways: *The Soul-utions*

Acknowledgements

I would like to express my sincerest gratitude to all my patients, through the years, for their stories and experiences which have added to the collective knowledge and inspiration of this book. I will always be indebted to Gary and Regina Siegel of The Linden Tree Healing Center in Poughkeepsie, New York, for giving me the first opportunity, way back then, to begin to work in the ways that created this book. I am especially indebted to Miranda Gray whose book, *The Red Moon*, provided a missing ingredient to my own understandings when it was first published and I thank her for her enlightening book. I have been honored to meet along the way some very special healers that, in their own unique ways, have shared their tools and added to my spiritual awareness. I am grateful to Marianne Collins for her kindness in introducing me to healing back in Poughquaq. I will always feel great admiration for the generous healers, Anne and Roger Warner, for their friendship, teachings and the comfort they brought to me in our time together in Shepton Mallet. I will never forget the support and nurturing I received from the dedicated healer, Ruth Bridgeman, in our work in Frome. I consider myself lucky to have been able to toss my hormonal woes and ideas at Susan Babilon through the years, who so kindly read the manuscript and gave her professional and female views in her very tactful way. The greatest gratitude goes to my husband, Keir Davidson, whose encouragement, love and belief has carried this book to fulfillment. With his gentle and caring hands he helped me see the logical structure of the book, while his healing presence provided the atmosphere to write it.

This Book is Dedicated to the Loving Memory of

My Mother
Ella

My Grandmothers
Susie and Ola

My Aunts
Viola and Judy

for their laughter and their pain
which has been instrumental
to my understanding

About the Author

Linda Crockett is a medical herbalist, nutritionist and healer, with a special interest in women's health, who has been working for 10 years as a holistic practitioner in the UK. Originally from Queens, New York, she received a bachelor's degree in nutrition from Queens College, City University of New York, in 1986, after careers on Wall Street and as a potter in upstate New York. Soon after graduating, she began studying herbal medicine which took her to England to study at the renowned School of Phytotherapy, later becoming a member of the National Institute of Medical Herbalists in England. With her interest, passion and research always in women's hormonal health, she started running holistic well women clinics in Somerset, England. Broadening her work and life with the study of healing, she became a member of the National Federation of Spiritual Healers in the UK which has been a turning point in her understanding of hormones and women's health. Besides running her private practice at The Stone House Healing Centre, on the Welsh/Shropshire border, Linda teaches Herbal Medicine, runs workshops and writes.

She can be contacted at lindacrockett@talktalk.net or
www.thestonehousehealingcentre.co.uk

Introduction

I am sitting in my office thinking about this book; the sun is pouring in on this clear warm morning. A slight breeze carries the scent of rose and honeysuckle through the open window. I can hear the wind moving through the pinewood on the hill above and see the circular flow of sheep passing single file around it. The sky is clear blue and full with buzzards circling rhythmically, their soft dolphin-like whispers punctuating the quiet calm. My eyes wander to the white and pink cosmos flowers alongside the gate. I am thinking about my 25 year journey to this place and hope I can bring all I have learned forward in a caring and inspiring way.

For many, the road to a peaceful existence often begins with what appears to be a negative impetus; something within that gnaws away at them, preoccupies their mind, motivates their decisions and becomes their obsession. This is just what happened to me and is the power behind this book. I suffered dramatically with premenstrual syndrome over the years and without its disturbing monthly reminders, the depressive episodes, the lethargic incapacities, the irrational outbursts, the explosive rages and the battles with weight, I would never have been so determined to make sense out of the chaos of hormones and their cyclical fluctuations. It was my frustrations with treatment and the inability for anyone to explain what was wrong with me that caused my initial need to take control and learn as much as I could about hormones. It was this wild premenstrual energy that fuelled me from one course and diploma to the next, and it was my desperation that kept bringing me to each new therapy, looking deeper within myself. From this I somehow managed, over the years, to develop a healthy lifestyle, loving relationship, successful career, and a more peaceful balance within myself. What I realize now is that I have become the therapist I wish I could have met back then, who could have given me the comfort and reassurance and, above all, the *soul-utions* I needed. But then again, had I met such a person I would have missed the experience of the healing journey I had to make.

From my own experience, and the last 10 years working with women as a holistic practitioner, I have become very familiar with the problems women face and the hormonal triggers behind so many of them. Women come to me as confused as I was, desperately trying to make sense of the diverse and complicated symptoms of premenstrual syndrome. Many turn up angered by the side effects they have developed from their use of synthetic hormones in treating endometriosis or menopause. Some come in frustrated with their increasing weight and appetite, remaining unaware of underlying conditions such as polycystic ovary syndrome or insulin resistance that maybe powering their inability to control their food intake. Then there are those that appear in my office tired and exhausted after failing to get their health practitioners to acknowledge or understand their problems with candida.

But you really cannot blame anyone. Hormones are tricky, and do not easily fit into the orderly, diagnostic world of medicine. There is a mystery surrounding hormones and women never quite seem to get the definitive answers they are hoping for. They get blood screenings, scans, swabs, scrapes and smears, the result of which all come back negative, while all along they know intuitively that something is wrong. Sometimes women are absolutely certain they are hypothyroid, but blood tests never substantiate their claim. Some women are sure their ravenous appetite is a blood sugar problem, but their glucose tolerance test does not give them the results they expected. Many women are puzzled by their cyclic return of vaginitis which never seems to show up in a swab but continues to cause them problems. Others throw their hands up in exasperation when thinking they have cured their tender breasts, period pains and thrush, only to have them return next cycle with a vengeance. Welcome to the baffling world of hormones.

We seem to be missing something important about hormones. Hormones do not exist solely on the physical level, but are an intricate part of the inner world of women. I believe most women intuitively know they have a hormonal problem, they just cannot get anyone else to believe them; and worse, they have begun doubting themselves. So when they call me, and start explaining their history and I agree and confirm their intuition, they are reassured and hopeful. I have come to believe that the chances are, they do have a hormonal problem, but it may not be the hormone everyone is looking for. In fact, not only are we looking for the wrong hormone, but many times we may be treating the wrong symptoms, possibly the wrong condition, and more importantly, probably missing most of the women behind the condition. This can mean that for many women the real cause of their problem is never identified and therefore never resolved. So much of treatment today is geared at the physical body and its symptoms, greatly reducing the possibilities of hormonal treatment and our perception of hormonal disease. What we are overlooking is that hormones, besides being a physical issue, are driven by the energy of emotions, and are guided by the inner spirit of women. If we ignore these other aspects we will never be able to balance our hormones or heal our lives.

The source of much of my inspiration and guidance for this book has come from my patients and the life stories they have generously shared with me. With each new consultation there came another story, and even though the details of the stories were always different, there remained a common thread in all of them. I began to see that preceding all hormonal conditions there was a history of stress: a stress caused by living a life which contained a longing to be loved, the cruelty of criticism, the despondency of loneliness, the hopelessness of poverty, the sadness of loss, the fear of rejection and the brutality of sexual abuse. These, I have come to believe, are the true origins of hormonal conditions: the traumas that cause the body's chemistry to change and what remain women's destructive unconscious wounds. It is these wounds that slowly undermine their belief in themselves and eventually take over as the dominating force, driving both their internal bodies and their lives in general. When self-beliefs are positive and life affirming, they bring health and happiness; when they are negative, a hopeless despair descends that acts as a powerful invitation to disease. When this point is reached, it is no longer a question of what they are eating or what their DNA holds, their despair will penetrate their body and soul, becoming a trigger of their hormone conditions. The messages the body receives are about how much women care about themselves, how much they love themselves, and how much they want to live. They may be able to fool the external world, but they cannot fool their internal world, disease is a manifestation of their hidden self-beliefs.

After years of working with women, I began to notice that there is a natural progression to healing, a way of moving us beyond our physical symptoms, down into our emotions, and then enabling entrance into our spiritual realm: a place that guides us into healing, forgiveness and understanding. It was a format I was unconsciously using in my work, the same I had used in my own healing and it seemed natural to use it as the structure of this book, so readers can progress through their own healing journey, reading through each chapter. Because hormonal conditions are surrounded by ambiguity and women do not always have the language or tools to explain them, we need a great deal of reassurance. In Chapter 1 this comes by acknowledging our hormonal symptoms and offering an approachable explanation of each hormone in the body, the glands they come from, and the endocrine system they are part of, creating the building blocks for the work ahead and providing a new confidence in the symptoms and the body. With an encouraging and positive relationship, we can proceed to Chapter 2 where we accept the energy behind emotions and its role in altering hormones. This often brings a sense of relief as we begin to recognize that our problems may be more about ourselves and our lives, rather than being simply a medical condition. Now empowered by a new sense of our own role in controlling our conditions, in Chapter 3 we can confront the unconscious beliefs we hold about ourselves, find the reasons for our broken spirits, the imbalances of our hormones and the disorder of our lives. With the enthusiasm that comes with understanding and a sense of control, we explore some healing tools in Chapter 4, hoping that in them we can find a better way to love and care for ourselves and find the *soul-utions* to our hormonal conditions. In Section II we look in detail at some of the most commonly misunderstood hormonal conditions I see in my practice, offering my holistic experience of each condition and some possible *soul-utions*. As you move through each chapter I hope you are stimulated by the knowledge of your body, intrigued by the energy of your emotions, and driven by the wisdom of your spirit along a path of self-healing.

I know I have tapped into something universal that women understand. During my workshops I see women nodding passionately in recognition; some have had a spontaneous and compelling urge to share their story, while others come to me afterwards holding my hands in gratitude, tears in their eyes. I have come to see these actions as an identification with their own intuitive feelings that I, somehow, am able to ignite in the depth of their unconscious mind: something they have always known but never had the tools, language or self-confidence to believe in. This book is about how to be able to access the knowledge that brings about true self-awareness and how to benefit from the wisdom that this understanding can offer.

Today my journey continues or, we could say, comes full circle. I started this journey as a young premenstrual woman and now in my 50s, the irony is that I have healed my premenstrual syndrome, but now I am menopausal. But with all I have learned, I now look forward to this age and all it will bring me. I no longer fear my body, or its cycles, and trust in its wisdom which has fuelled this book. It now carries me through my journey, in a place where I can watch the sheep pass through the pinewood each day, hear the wind through the trees, watch the buzzards circling in the sky and the clouds roll over the hills.

Chapter 1

The Physical

First Consultation

When a patient first arrives for their initial consultation there is always a great amount of anticipation. Women do not always know what to expect, so I make sure that when I open the door, they are greeted warmly and the room is comforting. They first notice the scent of geranium oil filling the room with a comforting ease, something that always brings a smile to their faces. The sound of American Indian flute music quietly plays in the background, adding a hypnotic rhythm to the room, while the soft warm lighting highlights the vase of pink roses, conveying an encouraging friendliness. Reassured by the atmosphere, their apprehension fades, sometimes there is even a visible sense of relief in their eyes, as their intuition confirms they have come to the right place.

When consultations gets underway, we begin to explore what is most on patients' minds and this is usually their physical symptoms. The physical is the easiest place to begin; it's the most accessible at the beginning of a therapeutic relationship and has the most urgent needs. It is the physical symptoms that make their days harder, keep their minds preoccupied, and which become the focus of their discomfort. There is usually an immediacy with physical symptoms, women are not initially interested in how these physical symptoms evolved, or what they mean to their life, all they want is relief from them. Women come in because they are fearful of having severe period pains during exams, their premenstrual tension is destroying their relationships, they have an insatiable appetite that ruins every hope of losing weight, their heavy bleeding is draining their energy, the hair on their upper lips is becoming more noticeable, they cannot eat certain foods like they use to, or their night sweats are preventing them from sleeping. They come in frustrated and distressed by the unpredictability of their symptoms, or by the constraints they impose, but most of all they come in because their physical symptoms are adding more stress to their lives making them unable to cope with anymore. I often hear an unconscious plea in women's voices, to free them from the burden and discomfort of their symptoms and to get them out of their lives. There is something about hormonal symptoms that scare women terribly: a sense of fear and unwillingness, even a resistance, to accept them as their own. Without being able to relate to their physical symptoms, women can become victims to them, losing their power to control them and their pains get stronger, fatigue greater, appetite more out of control and anxiety unpredictable. Some women come in so overwhelmed by their physical symptoms, they seem to have lost their identity to them and their self-image becomes based on them.

The unease which surrounds hormonal symptoms has a lot to do with the way they present themselves; sometimes symptoms show up in multiples and may often be coming from more than one organ. Even more unsettling, they may also affect emotions and alter moods. There may be loose bowels with itchy skin, aggression with night sweats, tender breasts accompanying fatigue, period pains along with anxiety, lethargy and a bloated belly, or depression following eating. Hormonal symptoms do not always make sense. They confuse women with their ambiguous origins, panic them with their erratic nature, shock them with their drama, and then mock them by coming back just when they thought they were gone for good. To make matters worse, when the hormones are tested, they inevitably come back normal, even though persistent symptoms clearly indicate a problem exists. In the end, women may be offered birth control pills, hormone replacement therapy or anti-depressants and they may be strongly tempted, because hormones can bring women to the point of desperation when they begin to question their own mental health. It is this desperation I hear in my patient's voices during consultations, not knowing where to turn and what to do.

There is a huge hole in the understanding of hormonal conditions. Some of this comes from the limitations in medicine today, focusing too heavily on the physical symptoms, reducing and compartmentalizing them to the extent that they no longer have any significance to the women, their cycles or their lives. Some of the blame must go to the aggressive promotion of synthetic hormones as the answer to hormonal conditions which has occurred in the last 30 years. If we go back further in history we can find an ingrained cultural negativity that developed over the centuries, in relation to women's bodies and their cycle. The long-term effect of all these has been to erode the control women have over their health, distance them from their bodies and remove them further from their female wisdom, which is their greatest asset when it comes to their health. The only way to fill this hole in hormonal health is to bring hormone knowledge back to women in a manner they respond to and in a way that sparks their intuitive wisdom. Women are often comforted by knowing the realities of their hormones, where their symptoms are coming from and why they may have occurred. Demystifying the physical symptoms of hormones brings an ease and reduces the fear surrounding them. I often see women leave consultations feeling confident and happier in themselves, an immediate change that I attribute to their sudden understanding of the true nature of their hormonal symptoms and the fact that they have much more control over them than they thought. I hope by the end of the chapter the reader will share something of this liberating sense of understanding.

The Endocrine System: *Home to Hormones*

Hormones are only a small portion of a very large network called the endocrine system. The intrigue of this system of the body is that it consists of many distinct glands, scattered widely throughout the body, apparently unrelated, but which never the less communicate and work as a whole. What gives these glands this ability to communicate with each other and work collectively as a group, even though distinct from one another is their messengers: the hormones. Through hormones, three tiny glands positioned together in the centre of the brain (the hypothalamus, the pituitary gland and the pineal gland), communicate with the thyroid gland in the neck, the thymus gland in the chest, the pancreas gland in the abdomen, the ovaries in the pelvic cavity, and the adrenal glands in the mid back to form the endocrine system, all working together to sustain life. Each gland performs a vital function through its manufacture of unique hormones which are released into the blood stream, carried to distant glands and tissues by carrier molecules and met by receptors that helps them locate and trigger their physiological response. Through the integration and communication of all these glands, hormones, carriers and receptors, some of the most important processes of the life are carried out: making of energy, sexual development, growth and repair of tissues, immunity to infections, digestion and assimilation of food, protection from stress and reproduction of the species.

It is the interaction of the glands in the endocrine system that maintain the crucial balance that enables the above processes to occur without interruption or interference and which create health and well-being. But what adds the real power and complexity to all this is the strong link that the endocrine system shares with other systems of the body. The brain, nervous system and immune system form an even broader association with the endocrine system, with information passing between each and influencing the workings of one another. Through this dynamic control, the workings of women's hormones become influenced not only by the internal interactions between the glands, but also by the alterations in brain activity, changes in nervous responses and modifications made by the immune system. Hormones fluctuate then, under the influence and response to their own internal rhythm, by the alterations in brain and nervous system chemicals called neurotransmitters, and from immune compounds released by the immune system. This means that the causes of many common hormonal conditions lie not only in the glands themselves, but also in the wider activity and health of these other systems.

With a network so intricately linked in communication and activity, if one gland begins to weaken and produce an inappropriate amount of hormone, it will inevitably affect the others, and in time, the whole system will be affected. The same can occur when either the nervous system or the immune system is overburdened by anxiety or illness, producing repercussions that filter through to the endocrine system. This situation creates one of the biggest dilemmas in the treatment of hormonal conditions: how to separate and treat the primary problem rather than secondary symptoms, and perhaps more concerning these days, how to avoid further disrupting an already dysfunctional endocrine system by taking synthetic hormones that will, in all likelihood, trigger further imbalances. Welcome to the world of hormones. This is the challenge today, and one which makes it essential that women understand the intricacies of the endocrine system and all its glands, hormones, carrier molecules, receptors and external links, so better decisions can be made when it comes to health. With this in mind, let us begin by building up a detailed understanding of each gland and start the process of removing some of the mystery and ambiguity from the world of hormones.

The Hypothalamus: *The Consolidator*

The hypothalamus is the gland where all these important connections occur. To be able to accommodate all this activity, the hypothalamus functions not only as a gland of the endocrine system, but also as an organ of the brain and a part of the nervous system. Through all of these functions, the hypothalamus becomes essential to the integrity and balance of women's hormones. As an organ of the brain, it coordinates and processes information received from the external world through the senses of sight, smell and hearing. It forms links with the higher parts of the brain, providing information about primal instinct, emotions, desire, sex, aggression and motivation. In responding to this brain activity, in its capacity as a gland, it sends out hormonal signals to the pituitary gland, enabling the necessary physiological changes to keep up with these ever-changing life experiences. In turn, it receives hormonal signals from the other glands, creating a circular pattern of information moving in and out of the hypothalamus. The last of the hypothalamus' important roles is to regulate the autonomic nervous system (a part of the nervous system which controls unconscious actions, those triggered without intent or thought, such as breathing, the beating of the heart, blinking of the eyes, movement of limbs, digestion and elimination). Through these combined functions, the hypothalamus balances the internal and external worlds of women and creates their stability.

For women, the information and energy that passes through the hypothalamus is what generates the cycles and rhythms of their lives. From it comes a female intelligence that starts puberty, instigates the menarche, maintains the menstrual cycle, enables ovulation and fertilization, prepares for pregnancy, supports through birthing, and knows when menopause should begin. The whole of women's life cycle and reproductive capability is consolidated in the hypothalamus, but this is also where these processes can become influenced by the health of the other glands, and on a wider level, the individual's emotions, stress levels, preoccupations and general health, all of this leaving them very open to interference and volatility. The hypothalamus channels this ever-changing mass of information through the pituitary gland and, in so doing so, exposes the other glands in the system to influences from women's everyday lives, an exposure which, in time, can alter their chemistry. As the hormones of the hypothalamus reach the pituitary gland there can be alterations in the texture of women's breasts and changes in how much water they retain. As these signals reach the other glands, the hypothalamus enforces both a direct and indirect influence over sleep patterns through the pineal gland, metabolism from the thyroid gland, infections with the thymus gland, appetite control at the pancreas gland, regularity of the menstrual cycle with the ovaries and the ability to cope with life's stresses from the adrenal glands. This is how women's lives have the ability to change hormonal balances and alter the physical body.

The Pituitary Gland: *The Organizer*

While the hypothalamus collects all this information, the pituitary gland helps organize and interpret it, converting it into physical responses which are then sent to all the associated glands and tissues. These include the thyroid gland, the adrenal glands, the ovaries, the breasts, skin and kidneys. This gives the pituitary gland an influence over many diverse and widespread functions of the body, which would normally not seem to have any relation to one another. It produces follicle stimulating hormone (FSH) and luteinizing hormone (LH) (the two hormones that control the release of estrogen and progesterone from the ovaries and make reproduction possible). From this gland comes human growth hormone (HGH), a hormone responsible for the growth and repair of all tissues, and for the development of female sexual characteristics such as breasts, body hair and the shaping of the female body through fat disposition. At the breast tissue level, the pituitary gland regulates prolactin, a hormone which enables milk production and breast feeding; while its hormone oxytocin maintains contractions of the breast in breast feeding and in the uterus at childbirth. Fluctuations in thyroid hormones are maintained through the pituitary gland, and energy and metabolism are controlled by its production of thyroid stimulating hormone (TSH). Through synthesis of adrenocorticotropic hormone (ACTH) it manages the amount of hormones produced in the cortex of the adrenal glands, governing stress hormones, sex hormones and water balance, with influences on blood sugar levels, mood and fertility. Antidiuretic hormone (ADH) is made in the pituitary gland, controlling blood volume and water balance, affecting the kidneys, blood vessels and the heart. At the skin level, it maintains pigmentation through the release of melanocytes stimulating hormone (MSH).

Although all these activities are unique in their own way, they are also intrinsically linked through the pituitary gland and anything that affects one of them will have repercussions on the others. Because of this, women often have more than one, sometimes seemingly unrelated hormonal symptom, occurring at the same time, confusing them as to its origin. One of the best examples of this is premenstrual syndrome, with its various symptoms of mood problems, breast tenderness, water retention, insatiable appetite and fatigue, all of which can arise through changes within the pituitary gland. In the same respect, women are often surprised to hear that their irregular cycles, heavy bleeding and infertility could have more to do with imbalances coming through the pituitary gland than from the ovaries themselves. In menopause, it could also be the pituitary gland that can be responsible for women having a variety of symptoms including high blood pressure, fatigue, anxiety, weight gain, breast tenderness, joint pain and loss of libido, none which seem to have a common root. This same variety of symptoms can be found in women taking birth control pills or hormone replacement therapy; upsetting the natural balance of the pituitary gland and possibly causing symptoms ranging from migraines, changes in skin pigmentation, raging appetites, weight gain, sluggishness and depression. Many common hormonal symptoms originate through the hypothalamus and pituitary gland but continue to be treated at the level of the ovaries, only complicating hormones further.

The Pineal Gland: *The Timekeeper*

The pineal gland is the last of the glands that make up the powerful threesome in the central brain. Its distinction from the hypothalamus and the pituitary gland is that it controls the rhythmic timing of biological processes, whether occurring hourly, daily, monthly or through the years. Through the hours, the pineal gland stimulates organs and hormones into activity. Daily, it controls the sleep pattern. Monthly, it manages the fluctuation of hormones in the menstruation cycle and through the years it influences the timing of menarche and menopause. This ability to program time and create rhythm is made possible by the pineal gland's unique characteristic of being light sensitive. As light passes through the eyes, activation of these rhythms and cycles occur through coordination with the hypothalamus, pituitary gland and nervous system. It is believed to be changes in the intensity of moonlight which stimulate the pineal gland into sending its signals to the hypothalamus to initiate changes in women's cycles; this shadowy but inescapable link explains the moon's importance as a symbol of fertility through the centuries and the strong, instinctual attachment many women feel with the moon but find difficult to articulate.

This interesting ability of the pineal gland to react to light is supported by the nervous system, which supplies it with the neurotransmitter, serotonin (one of the stimulating neurotransmitters which keep the central nervous system active). From serotonin, the pineal gland builds its own hormone, melatonin (the hormone which makes all light sensitive reactions possible and which has a strong affect on women and their cycles). Normally, in daylight, serotonin levels are high in the pineal gland, creating a state of wakefulness, but as darkness comes the pineal gland begins using up the serotonin, converting it into melatonin, which in turn encourages sleep. This efficient sleep pattern is, however, vulnerable to the natural reductions in serotonin levels that occur just prior to menstruation each cycle and during menopause and can cause disruption in the normal sleep patterns at these times. This can result in wakefulness similar to that which some women experience during a full moon; when the bright moonlight reduces the conversion of serotonin to melatonin and they find themselves wide awake, alert and stimulated, after only a few hours sleep. Seasonally, some women are susceptible to a physical and mental sluggishness when the darker mornings and shorter days of autumn decrease the amount of serotonin available at the pineal gland, leaving them with the uncomfortable symptoms of seasonal affective disorder (SAD). But for most women, the pineal gland's production of melatonin becomes even more influential through its role in the timing of their menstrual cycle. Historically, the lack of light during the dark moon encouraged more melatonin to be made, initiating the release of hormones from the hypothalamus and stimulating the pituitary gland into releasing follicle stimulating hormone (FSH) and luteinizing hormone (LH), which brought about the start of a new cycle. This used to cause many women to bleed most often around dark moons and ovulate most often with the coming of a full moon. But today, with the huge increase of ambient lightening from streets and homes making moon light less significant, there has been more interference with the pineal gland's conversion of serotonin to melatonin, causing more disruptions in women's rhythms, their menstrual cycle, and their fertility. Sadly, this also diminishes their intuitive sense of attachment to the moon and its rhythms, and with it the comfort and affirmation that this deep connection to the greater world outside themselves can bring.

The Thyroid: *The Energizer*

The thyroid gland is the first gland that we find outside the brain, sitting instead in a central position in the neck from where it can target all the body's cells, either upward into the brain, or downward into the body. Its hormones Triiodothyronine (T3) and thyroixine (T4) act as accelerators for the life-sustaining processes within the body's cells, known as metabolism. How competent these hormones are at performing these cellular processes determines how efficiently oxygen is utilized, food is digested, waste is excreted, tissues are repaired, information is processed in the brain and energy is created. The accumulative efforts of all of these cellular processes provides our physical and mental vitality. Through them, the thyroid gland is responsible for the regulation of body weight, the development of sexual organs, how accurately the body's temperature is maintained, how much cholesterol is excreted, how easy it is to learn new things, and how energetic we feel. Overall, the thyroid gland's position means that it exerts a huge influence on the health and well-being of women. This is confirmed by looking at the thyroid gland's two most common disorders, hypothyroidism and hyperthyroidism, both having long lists of symptoms associated with them affecting women at many levels, including their mental concentration, skin condition, eye strength, hearing ability, sinuses drainage, voice quality, heart function, bone strength, quality of blood, health of teeth and gums, bowel regularity, cholesterol levels and reproduction.

The encompassing control the thyroid has over the body and mind comes through the strong connections it has with the hypothalamus, pituitary gland, ovaries, adrenals glands and the liver, all of which give it a powerful influence on hormonal health. The amount of thyroid hormone produced is directed by the hypothalamus and all of its links, and influenced by the activity of the pituitary gland, which sends out thyroid stimulating hormone (TSH). In terms of menstrual health, this leaves the thyroid gland function open to the same interferences that affect the glands in the brain and can generate many common menstrual problems including irregular cycles, erratic bleeding, fertility problems, weight and appetite issues, fatigue, anxiety, extreme body temperatures, night sweats, sleep disturbances and changes in mood. The thyroid hormones are also susceptible to changes in the levels of estrogen, progesterone and testosterone, as they all vie for the same carriers and receptors, so imbalances in one will affect the other. In conditions where estrogen levels may be elevated (as in endometriosis, insulin resistance, candida and breast disease), in premenstrual syndrome (where progesterone levels may be low) and in cases of polycystic ovary syndrome (where testosterone levels could be high), the performance of thyroid hormones may be hindered. This can often make women feel as if they have hypothyroidism, although the thyroid gland is producing normal levels of hormones; one of the inconsistencies which occurs frequently in thyroid hormone blood screening. The liver can also be a source of thyroid dysfunction in women where viruses, drugs, medication, alcohol or illness cause reduced liver function, also reducing its ability to convert thyroid hormone T4 to T3. These situations often cause thyroid gland dysfunction to be misunderstood and confused, preventing women from getting the care and treatment they need. Where the thyroid gland is concerned, it is best to consider women's full hormonal profile and liver function to get a broader picture of their endocrine health, rather than simply concentrating on their thyroid hormone levels alone.

The Thymus Gland: *The Protector*

The thymus gland is another of the glands that performs a double task. Besides being an endocrine gland, it also functions as an important lymphatic organ. Made up of tissue derived from the immune system, the thymus gland serves the endocrine system as a powerful protector against illness. It is unique among the glands in that, instead of growing and developing through puberty as the others do, it does the opposite and reduces in size. It is largest during infancy and childhood, which may help explain its function in providing immune protection during an age that is vulnerable to illnesses and which can impede a child's development into adulthood. When growth is complete in late adolescence, it decreases in size, but continues to work as an ally of the immune system. Its most important hormone, thymosin, assists in the transformation of white blood cells into T cells (the cells that fight infections and keeps abnormal growths in check). Conditions linked with a low functioning thymus gland are those associated with immune dysfunction such as allergies, especially, asthma, hay fever and eczema, and those which are considered autoimmune, where the immune system fails to recognize its own tissue and begins working against itself instead (as seen in myasthenia gravis and lupus). Other conditions linked to the thymus gland are those having to do with its neighboring organs, the lungs, heart and breasts, as they all share strong nerve and lympathtic connections. This increases the risks of pneumonia, congestive heart disease and cystic breast disease, if the thymus gland is weakened.

The protective nature of the thymus gland offers women an added security that helps sustain them in their reproductive role, and brings to the endocrine system an important link to the immune system. Women who have a genetic susceptibility to hormonal conditions do not always progress into full-blown cases because the thymus gland provides an immunity within the structure of the endocrine system that can prevent progression of these conditions. When the thymus gland is weakened by a poor diet, toxicity or stress, and its hormones not performing their immune responsibilities as they should, low level hormonal conditions can progress into chronic inflammatory conditions such as rheumatoid arthritis, fibromyaglia, chronic fatigue syndrome and candida. The efficiency of the thymus gland should be questioned when there are unusual growths in the reproductive organs like endometriosis and fibroids. Although these are conditions of the womb, the thymus gland should be capable of producing immune compounds that prevent these abnormal growths from occurring. The same scenario can be seen in some breast and lung cancers, with their close proximity to the thymus gland and their shared lympathtic and nerve connections. This gives the opportunity for cancers to spread easily through these channels without the full protection of a functioning thymus gland. After giving birth, when the reserves of women are lowered, and the thymus gland is less efficient, it may make women more susceptible to infections in the breast and perineum. Chronic viral infections, like glandular fever and herpes, can continue to cause problems through the lifetime without the help and support of this protecting gland. It's not a gland often associated with women's hormone health, but one which carries huge implications.

The Pancreas: *The Balancer*

Where the thyroid gland helps make energy, the pancreas provides the raw material in the form of glucose. Through its control over digestion, the pancreas assists the breakdown of carbohydrates, producing its elemental component, glucose. From the uptake of glucose into cells, energy is made and life sustained. Although the body can also get energy from the breakdown of proteins and fat, it is carbohydrates which provide the fastest source of energy. When cells need energy, they need it immediately and cannot wait for the next meal, so in order to survive, humans have evolved with a way of keeping a constant level of glucose in the blood for all energy needs, whether food comes regularly or not. This critical level of glucose is what is called blood sugar and is held in the blood stream, as in a holding pen, until it is needed by the cells. The pancreas maintains the appropriate amount of blood sugar through its two hormones, insulin and glucagon. Insulin lowers blood sugar after a meal by physically carrying it into the cells, while glucagon raises blood sugar by breaking down stored fat or lean tissue and replenishing the blood sugar levels when food intake is insufficient to meet energy needs. Through the actions of these two hormones, a steady and balanced blood sugar should be provided for all energy needs.

Because reproduction is highly dependent on a carefully controlled blood sugar, the pancreas and its hormones are strongly related to estrogen and progesterone levels, all having the capacity to affect blood sugar. Many women may recognize the subtle, and sometimes not so subtle, changes that occur in their blood sugar levels through their menstrual cycle and its fluctuating hormones. The week after bleeding, estrogen levels rise to the highest levels of the cycle, helping to rebuild a new womb lining. The needs are great for this activity and high estrogen levels provide the increase in metabolism to sustain this extensive restoring process, while also improving the ability of insulin to move glucose into the cells so that the blood sugar is more efficiently maintained. This gives women much more control over their appetite and brings more balance to their lives since they experience less hunger, fewer food cravings, make better food choices, feel less full and have more energy during this phase. This all changes when estrogen lowers and progesterone becomes dominate during the luteal phase. Progesterone naturally slows the ability of insulin to get glucose into cells as it is the hormone of pregnancy and begins to conserve blood sugar in its preparation for conception. This causes the cells to feel less satisfied with the amount of glucose they are getting, delaying the satiety signal to brain, while the blood sugar is teeming with glucose. What follows is a common premenstrual episode for many women where their appetite is greatly increased, strong food cravings occur for fast burning foods like carbohydrates, there is fatigue and lethargy afterwards, causing even more cravings for stimulants, like chocolate, to keep energy and mood up, producing the highs and lows of blood sugar. The women who feel these changes most dramatically are those with a diet high in carbohydrates, those with polycystic ovary syndrome, or those using contraception, all of which can intensify this natural fluctuation in blood sugar and cause more uncomfortability. At these times, when the blood stream is more full with glucose, women become more susceptible to an overgrowth of fungus and can lead to thrush, food intolerances, irritable bowel syndrome, migraines, skin irritations, premenstrual syndrome, depression, anxiety and palpitations during this part of their cycle. Over the years the dangerous combination of high levels of estrogen and insulin can increase the risk of cancer of the breast and uterus in susceptible women. Blood sugar is a vital aspect in women's hormonal health and well-being and any interference in the functioning of the pancreas gland only adds to women's hormonal burden.

The Ovaries: *The Life Givers*

All of the unfertilized eggs that women are born with and which give them their great potential to create life, are stored within the ovaries. Women's lives silently revolve around the patterns of change which occur each month to encourage these eggs to become fertilized. In doing so, the ovaries produce their two important hormones, estrogen and progesterone, which make women uniquely female and which make life possible. While estrogen ensures the body is prepared and ready for repro-duction, progesterone supports it through conception and pregnancy. It is through the differentiated activities of estrogen and progesterone, with their individual attributes and alternating domination, that the menstrual cycle is created and divided into its four phases referred to as the menstrual phase, follicular phase, ovulation phase and luteal phase. Each of these phases has its own specific goal that is directed by its individual hormone pattern, all creating the cyclic nature of women. The menstrual phase is a time when all ovarian hormones are low, facilitating the shedding of the old womb lining and signaling the hypothalamus to start another cycle through its release of gondotrophic releasing hormone (GnRH). This acts as a signal to the pituitary gland to release FSH, and begins the start of the follicular phase by stimulating the ovaries to bring forward one of their unfertilized follicles for development into an egg. As the egg develops during this phase, it produces increasing amounts of estrogen, which begins to rebuild the womb lining. Once the egg is fully developed, its hormone production causes a surge of luteinizing hormone (LH) to be released from the pituitary gland, initiating ovulation with the fertile egg breaking away from the ovarian follicle and moving up the fallopian tube to await the arrival of sperm. In the luteal phase the remaining follicle metamorphoses into a hormone producing gland called the corpus luteum, which produces estrogen and progesterone and will prepare the womb for conception. If conception does not occur, the corpus luteum degenerates and levels of hormones decline, a signal to the hypothalamus to begin the cycle again.

It is the interactions between the hypothalamus and the pituitary gland that support the ovaries' extraordinary ability to create life and maintain the menstrual cycle, but it is also within these links that the risks of menstrual irregularities are greatly increased. Dysfunctions in the other glands and changes in a women's nervous response or immune function, all filter back through the hypothalamus and pituitary gland, changing the signals to the ovaries. This leaves each phase of the menstrual cycle open to a variety of possible disturbances that can affect levels of estrogen and progesterone and the regularity of the menstrual cycle. For example, the menstrual phase is open to extremes in blood flow when there is dysfunction in the thyroid gland, some women having an abnormally heavy flow and some with unusually light flow. Through periods of stress or trauma, both the hypothalamus and the adrenal glands can instigate changes that impede the follicle developing during the follicular phase, causing women to experience irregular cycles or stop menstruating altogether. The small peak in hormones which initiate ovulation can be interrupted by abnormal insulin levels from the pancreas causing ovulation pains, ovarian cysts, failure to ovulation, and the possibility of a day or so of premenstrual-like feelings around ovulation. The dominance of progesterone during the luteal phase, normally causes a slight lowering of the immune response, which in some women can increase the risk of thrush, vaginitis, water retention, breast tenderness, aches, pains, and gum and teeth problems during this phase. The competence of the ovaries and the cycle is a good indicator of the overall health and well-being of women, and whatever health issues are occurring elsewhere in the body will eventually makes their way into the cycle through the encompassing nature of the endocrine system.

The Adrenal Glands: *The Defenders*

The adrenal glands have a powerful influence on women's hormonal health, through their connections with both the nervous system and the ovaries. It is through these that the adrenal glands perform the difficult task of normalizing body functions no matter how much change, danger and stress there is in women's lives. To support this extraordinarily complex task, the adrenal glands are divided into two distinct parts, the medulla and the cortex, each with their individual hormones, unique functions and tissue composition, which enable them to reach and affect different parts of the body. The medulla is made up of the same tissue as the nervous system and acts as a branch of the autonomic nervous system called the sympathetic nervous system. Under the control of the sympathetic nervous system physiological processes such as breathing, pumping of the heart, circulation of the blood and movement of the limbs occurs automatically without thought or intent. In emergencies, the medulla is able to change these activities to preserve life through its production of the stress hormones, adrenalin and noradrenalin. The inner cortex, on the other hand, is made up of tissue related to that in the ovaries and produces hormones similar in structure and function to the sex hormones: estrogen, progesterone, and testosterone. It also produces the important stress hormone, cortisol, which unlike the other stress hormones has more sustaining results. The other hormone produced in the cortex is aldosterone which controls water and mineral balance through the kidneys. All the hormones of the adrenal glands have the power and reach to affect all parts of the body when there is stress, disrupting hormonal balance and imparting a powerful influence on the development of hormonal conditions in women.

The actions of the adrenal glands help promote the preservation of life, but the abuse or overuse of these glands also has the potential to destroy life. Continuous stress in women's lives cause output of excessive stress hormones, changing the chemistry of the body and affecting the stability of women. Through the stimulation of adrenalin, women get the extra energy and strength they need to keep them functioning during troubled times. However, it can also bring with it an uncomfortable sense of anticipation, with them always expecting the worse to happen as their body is pumped up by adrenalin and generates anxiety, restlessness, agitation, panic attacks and high blood pressure when it continues for too long. Noradrenalin provides women under threat with protection by increasing circulation of blood flow to the brain and heart, keeping them alert, focused and ready for an emergency. But if blood is shifted away from the lower body to meet the demands of the upper body for too long, it leaves the lower joints in the hips, knees and feet more open to chronic inflammation conditions like arthritis. However, the greatest damage to women and hormones comes from cortisol, produced when women live with stress on a more regular basis. When cortisol is released its actions are beneficial, enabling survival under threat, but if its actions continue for too long they become destructive, especially on the reproductive hormones. As both cortisol and progesterone are made from the same cholesterol building block, too much cortisol production can reduce progesterone levels and be a factor in premenstrual syndrome. The increase in cortisol, in relationship to other hormones, also saturates the limited hormone carriers and receptors, reducing the ability of other hormones to elicit their responses properly. This is sometimes the case in polycystic ovary syndrome, where testosterone - unable to find free carrier molecules - flows unattached through a woman's blood stream causing male-patterned hair growth. Without enough receptors for aldosterone, water retention and breast tenderness can occur in women, while also obstructing normal mineral metabolism in the kidneys, leaving women more at risk of developing osteoporosis. Cortisol further compromises hormonal balance by reducing the liver's ability to break down estrogen completely, causing higher estrogen levels in the blood. The combination of high estrogen and a reduced production of progesterone, generate what is called estrogen dominant conditions, where the important balance between estrogen and progesterone is lost and estrogen flows through the blood stream, sometimes without carrier molecules and sometimes unable to attach to receptors. This can be the cause of over-stimulation of reproductive tissue as seen in endometriosis, fibroids, uterus and breast cancer. During menopause women may also find that if the adrenal glands are overworking to make cortisol, they may not be able to efficiently produce enough estrone, the estrogen that takes over in menopause and which prevents many of the uncomfortable hot flushes, night sweats, insomnia, fatigue, vaginal dryness and lowered libido. Many common hormonal problems that are thought to be issues of the reproductive organs can often have their start within the adrenal glands when stress is involved, something that will become clearer in the following chapters.

Conclusion

Women usually leave the first consultation feeling they have a better understanding of their physical symptoms and with this comes reassurance. Much of the fear and anxiety surrounding hormonal conditions is centered around their ambiguity; simply making hormones and glands more understandable can, in itself, bring a peace of mind. They may go away with a herbal remedy or some diet advice to help ease their symptoms, but most importantly, they leave understanding their hormonal condition more, bringing them a greater sense of control in its management. For some women this is enough and they go away more confident in their bodies and relieved of their discomforts, not needing to go any further. But there are others that may have recognized, through the consultation, that there is something beyond their physical symptoms that needs to be addressed in order for true healing to occur, and they may decide to come back for a second consultation. From there we can move away from the physical symptoms, putting more emphasis on the women themselves, in the hope that they will help reveal the real cause of their hormonal conditions.

Chapter 2

The Emotional

Second Consultation

I always feel fortunate when women return for a second consultation, as it gives us an opportunity to work more deeply and produce more lasting results. Coming to this consultation they are now comfortable with the understanding of their physical symptoms and walk in with an enthusiastic anticipation for what may arise next. As we begin, I am looking for an opening to emerge where the origins of their symptoms become more obvious. The room is set to allow this to occur with the clarifying aromas of pine and cedar wood oils warming in the burner, bringing their resinous earthiness to the room. The soft sound of Icelandic music plays in the background, filling the room with gentle tones that make the space feel more secure. A warm yellow light from a globular lamp creates an intimacy in the room. As we sit down, our eyes are drawn to the vivid purple African violets sitting between us.

With the formalities of the first meeting over, the patients become more comfortable with the therapeutic relationship and more willing and determined to find answers to their hormonal conditions. I have found, over the years, that women intuitively know what is wrong with them, they just need a gentle nudge in the right direction to bring it out. Many times they surprise themselves with the answer. I begin by exploring the period of time when they first noticed their physical symptoms. Usually this connects them to a memory of a stressful, sad or traumatic time in their lives, a time they would rather not remember and one they may have successfully blocked. I have begun to feel that physical symptoms take over when the memory has been repressed; possibly as a way of keeping the unconscious from fading. This way the body is reminded there is something that needs to be dealt with, even though they have removed it from their conscious mind. When women reconnect to this memory there are usually tears, or down cast eyes, as the memory comes flooding back. Then after a moment, there is a smile as they acknowledge the relationship between the two events, some even recall fleeting moments when they recognized this relationship themselves. Instincts are not always given the recognition they deserve, it could be women don't trust themselves enough to give them any thought, or maybe there is too much pain involved in going where they lead.

Women often tell me they would prefer their hormonal conditions to have a physical cause rather than an emotional one. They would like to believe their premenstrual syndrome is caused by a deficiency of vitamin B6 in their diet, rather than the stress from their job. There is relief in knowing that their weight is due to a sluggish metabolism rather than munching away their depression. It's a relief to hear their polycystic ovary syndrome is part of their inheritance instead of being a residue of their dysfunctional family. It helps to feel that a difficult menopause has more to do with hormones than the painful relationships they have had. There are many ways to justify physical symptoms and make them appear medically sound, and I find that women do it all the time. They do not want to believe they are carrying around the remnants of their life traumas and they are still causing them harm and controlling their lives, for that would seem a burden too big to bear.

Underlying many hormonal conditions is an emotional energy that powers their progression and distorts their symptoms. Although women may have bad diets, have a genetic tendency for an illness, are not getting enough sleep or are drinking and smoking too much, it does not automatically mean they will get ill. There is often something else going on that is more powerful than diet, can defy genetics and override lifestyle. Through the combined workings of the endocrine system, nervous system and immune system, a resistance is generated that reduces the impact of these factors. All women need to do to access this internal protection is to give their body the appropriate messages, letting them know that they want and deserve this special treatment. Unfortunately, this does not always happen and the messages the body receives are often contradictory and unclear. When life experiences make women doubt themselves, stop loving themselves, or stop believing in themselves, the messages these systems receive is weakened. There is less optimism, more despondency and the emotions become more powerful and destructive. As girls grow into women and their lives become more emotionally complicated, the messages they send their body can change from a spontaneous vitality in childhood to a cautious hesitation in adolescent, and as they move into womanhood the joint efficiency of these systems diminish allowing bad eating habits to slowly begin to cause toxicity, genetic predispositions becomes more apparent, and women beginning to find they can no longer abuse their bodies and get away with it.

It's All in Their Story

There is a long and slow development of hormonal conditions that can start in the early days after birth and continue through life. All women have a story and within it can be found the seeds that can develop into hormonal conditions. The stories may involve a longing to be loved by an elusive parent, a parent who is more needy than loving, or parents gripped by alcohol, drugs, nerves, or memories. Sometimes death or loss leave a lingering grief, in others there may have been a temper that had no limits. Some carry a big hole that adoption never filled, while others carry the dark secrets surrounding sexual abuse. These often occur in young girls' lives, around the same time they are building their own self-image through a process of observing and absorbing the reactions they generate in those they interact with, whether within or outside their immediate family. Unfortunately, neither family nor peer relationships are always healthy and children do not always get it right, fostering issues which go unresolved and then, in later life, quietly wear down a women's sense of well-being, leaving them depressed, repressed, frustrated, and angry, preventing them from living to their full potential. They soon find ways of coping and types of behavior that enable them to muddle through life. Often this behavior is negative, like biting nails, excessive hand washing, bullying peers, shoplifting, excessive dieting, drinking, drugs, and sexual promiscuity. These provide an outlet for the emotional stress they feel inside and hide the true cause of their unhappiness. The outcome of this early negative behavior is that it uses up enormous amounts of energy and becomes physically and emotionally draining. Not only does it make young women emotionally vulnerable, but it can also be the start of a physical change in their chemistry from which hormonal conditions can evolve later in their lives.

Emotions: *How Issues Get into Tissues*
The fuel behind this negative behavior is negative emotion. The emotional pain felt by some young girls when allowed to remain repressed, becomes a raw energy within their bodies; a wild energy locked within the cells, interfering and confusing their normal biological processes. Negative emotions are not easy to get rid of. Notice how easily they can be recalled by an innocent trigger, coming up with a vengeance, that is hard to put down again. Emotions need to be processed and often the way women react is by blocking them from their conscious thoughts so they can get on with their lives. This does not mean the emotions are gone, it just means they are hidden in a place where they can interfere and block the energy of life and slowly predispose women to hormonal imbalances and illness without them being

aware of it. Sometimes these emotions are there for a few months, sometimes a few years, and sometimes a whole lifetime. Women usually show you where they are holding their emotions during the consultation. Sometimes they sit hunched over, their drooping shoulders trying to shield their broken heart. Some sit covering their stomach, trying to hide their insecurity. Some sit nervously, maneuvering from one side to the other, trying hard to guard their sorrows. Others constantly clear their throat trying to hold back what they really want to say. While others move their glaze round and round the room, anywhere to avoid looking directly into my eyes. They do not want me to see the depth of their pain.

Women sometimes fool themselves, thinking the past is over and done with and they have moved on. Then one day, some silly incident occurs that triggers an ugly, irate and uncontrollable fury from within. It's totally out of character; an outburst so powerful they frighten themselves, and are left feeling ashamed by their actions. It may have been the way someone said something, it could have been a facial expression, or maybe a wave of the hand that set them off. It's like sticking a needle in a balloon; emotions are energy that generate an explosion when they go unexpressed. Repression gives emotions power, the longer they sit, the longer they fester, the more uncontrollable they become and the more destruction and illness they bring.

Emotions are a huge stress to the body, using up enormous amounts of energy and giving nothing back in return, other than unhappiness. In order for women to live under the stress of emotions, their bodies have to adapt and compensate. The chemical changes that occur to meet these demands are especially damaging to young girls, at a time in their lives when their bodies are trying to build strong links between their developing reproductive system, nervous system and immune system. This is the important network that will carry them through life and create their hormonal health and well-being. When emotional stress interferes with this essential stage in their development, they are left more susceptible to hormonal irregularities, mental and emotional disturbances, and immune deficiencies. Then as they get older and have to deal with demanding jobs, raise families, care for aging parents, cope with the death of loved ones, and the sadness of relationship breakdowns, they may begin to find their anxiety brings on candida, their shame leads to insulin resistance, their depression brings up premenstrual syndrome, their anger develops into polycystic ovary syndrome, their sadness turns into endometriosis and their grief increases hot flushes at menopause. If women do not take the time and try to understand their emotional triggers, or find ways to reduce the stresses of their daily lives, they may find themselves open to the havoc hormones can bring and may become victims to them.

The Endocrine System: *The Processing of Emotions*

It is through the endocrine system that negative emotions get processed and passed on to the physical body, becoming as much a part of women as their blood and bones. Negative emotions are generated in the brain upon external stimulation from what is seen, heard and felt. The limbic brain, also called the emotional center of the brain, become highly charged and forwards nerve impulses that alter brain chemistry through changes in neuro-transmitters, the chemical messengers of the brain. These changes are instantaneously transmitted to the hypothalamus where they get translated into physiological changes through the autonomic nervous system, enabling the body to cope with the new situation, even if it is threatening and unstable. Nerve impulses are also forwarded directly from the limbic brain down into the glands themselves through the extensive nerve pathways that exist between them. Through these routes, emotions are able to change the workings of the physical body. Fear, anger, sadness, shame and grief then become the initiators of change in the endocrine system and the origins of many common hormonal conditions. To better understand the influence emotions have on women's hormones, it is essential to understand the stress response, the process by which the endocrine system copes with stress and alters women's chemistry.

The Stress Response

As was briefly mentioned in the last chapter, the stress response is a set of biological processes occurring in the endocrine system that help ensure the body keeps functioning during periods of short or long term stress. This protective mechanism works through the hypothalamus which manages it, the autonomic nervous system which makes the necessary physiological changes, and the adrenal glands which produce the stress hormones that generate the results. It starts when danger is perceived in the limbic brain which then forwards a nerve impulse to the hypothalamus, exciting the sympathetic nervous system, the part of the autonomic nervous system that stimulates the body to deal with the danger at hand. Through the sympathetic nervous system, a cascade of stimulating reactions involving the hypothalamus, pituitary and adrenal glands occurs changing the chemistry of the body. When acute stress is perceived, the sympathetic nervous system sends out the stress hormones, adrenaline and noradrenalin from the adrenal medulla, providing the person with all the courage and energy they need to fight the threat or the power to flee from it, often called 'fight or flight'. To generate the extra energy that this type of crisis calls for, the stress hormones slow the everyday functions of digestion, urination and reproduction and redirects the energy and blood supply to those functions coping with the immediate emergency. The heart starts pumping faster to supply more blood, the brain becomes sharp and alert to focus on the task, the muscles become pumped with enough energy in case they need to run, and the blood stream fills with glucose to supply all the energy to meet these extreme demands, all occurring at a cost to normal metabolism. It is a reaction that evolved to help short-term stress, but for women who continue to live with emotional stress in their lives, the continual stimulation of these hormones can slowly bring on anxiety, restlessness, insomnia, digestive problems, heart complications, exhaustion, and hormonal conditions.

Because the heightened metabolism that adrenalin and noradrenalin produce is hard to sustain long-term, there is another adaptation of the stress response which occurs when the limbic brain perceives a more constant threat. To provide a more sustaining energy, the hypothalamus is stimulated into sending out corticotrophin releasing hormone (CRH) a hormone that signals the pituitary gland to release adrenocortropin (ACTH). Through ACTH the cortex of the adrenal glands are stimulated into releasing the stress hormone cortisol into the blood stream to supplement the energy supply needed for stresses that last months and years. With this comes, not only, the energy reserves and physiological changes to enable the body to cope with long-term stress, but also health consequences that affect women and their hormones. The actions of cortisol work by redistributing the energy contained within tissues to the areas of need. It does this by selectively breaking down tissue to release the energy and protein within, which can then be used to increase blood supply, accelerate breathing, and to supply more glucose for the extra energy needs. Although this mechanism benefits metabolism under long-term stress, if relied upon through the years, cortisol's actions can become degenerative, exhausting and can lead to disease. It takes away from the repairing and restoring processes of the body, and redirects all energy into degrading tissues. It drains the immune system, leaving it less able to provide the protection it should and alters the neurotransmitters, making one feel unsteady and vulnerable. But as seen in the last chapter, the production of cortisol changes hormone balance on many different levels, leaving women open to many common hormonal conditions.

When stress starts early in young girls' lives they are more at risk to the damaging affects of cortisol, not only for what it does to hormone balance, but also how it affects their immune system, digestion and metabolism. One of the earlier indications of cortisol overuse in young girls can be the start of inflammatory illnesses such as asthma, hay fever, eczema, a sign that their adrenal glands and the immune system are no longer able to mask these genetic tendencies any further. As the immune function becomes weakened by the production of cortisol, deep-seated infections, such as chronic fatigue syndrome and glandular fever, may be able to establish themselves. With its ability to change blood chemistry, cortisol may also be implicated in some cases of anemia and leukemia. Through its actions on the pancreas, cortisol can raise blood sugar levels to the extent that candida and thrush can thrive unhindered, while increasing the risks of obesity, insulin resistance and Type II diabetes in stressed women. With the liver having to do most of the tissue breakdown for cortisol, it can weaken liver function, while also placing a heavy burden on the elimination organs, especially the kidneys, which have to process the nitrogen waste produced. This can leave girls open to kidney infections and older women at risk of high blood pressure. With an excessive breakdown of fat occurring to provide energy, more fat molecules are released into the blood stream increasing the possibility of high cholesterol levels, arteriosclerosis, stroke and thrombosis. There can also come a time when the continual use of cortisol causes the adrenal glands to become exhausted by its production, reducing their ability to keep stress at bay and making women feel overwhelmed by all the changes around them. This can lead to the fatigue and illness of adrenal exhaustion and is often the cause of many hormonal conditions. In returning to the glands now, we can more fully appreciate how the stress response affects each one of them individually.

The Transforming Hypothalamus

Just as the hypothalamus maintains physical equilibrium, it is also responsible for emotional stability. Through its regulation of the autonomic nervous system, the hypothalamus is where emotions perceived in the brain are transformed into hormonal responses that can then interact with and influence the physical body. It is in this way that feelings and emotions come to exert a powerful, but often a detrimental force behind the physical processes of breathing, pumping of the heart, muscle contractions, movement of limbs, sleeping, digestion and hormone regulation. When the hypothalamus receives a nerve impulse from the brain (due to fear, anger, sadness or grief), it initiates physiological changes through the sympathetic nervous system that can modify, and even alter these processes. Although they are emotional responses, they have physical affects, some of which are more familiar and occur more immediately, like the wrinkling of the forehead, a lump in the throat, a flutter in the heart or a butterfly in the stomach, all of which are elicited by the stimulation of the sympathetic nervous system and which generates increased muscle tension. These are good examples of just how emotional stress turns into physical sensations. When these occur occasionally, tension resolves itself soon afterwards and the body returns to normal functioning. But if women's lives become subject to emotional stresses sustained over long periods, the affects can be more damaging, creating a physical tension that begins to be more permanent. This is the tension that produces emotional blocks and from which illness originates, not only generating tense shoulders, stiff necks, tightness in the chest and nervous stomachs, but also restricting the flow of life force and holding women back physically and emotionally.

As emotional stress is filtered down through the hypothalamus it affects, not only the glands and the physical body, but it can also change the woman's nervous response. As cortisol levels rise in women with stressed lives, the hypothalamus promotes alterations in the nervous system's neurotransmitters, serotonin, dopamine, noradrenalin and the endorphins. These are the chemicals essential for the feeling of well-being and have an enormous impact on how well women respond to and cope with the world around them. They help keep women focused, alert, lively and content when their levels are normal, but when they are disrupted, due to excessive cortisol, women can become agitated, tired, despondent and depressed. With each gland sensitive to specific neurotransmitters, any change in them can generate emotional and physical disturbances distinctive to each gland. As negative emotions and stress change the nerve impulses of the hypothalamus, neurotransmitters change too, leading to abnormal responses from the major glands: from the pituitary gland can come an irritable moodiness, from the pineal gland a great sadness, from the thyroid gland an intense sensitivity, from the thymus gland enormous grief, from the pancreas a wild instability, from the ovaries an intense volatility, and from the adrenal glands a terrible apprehension. It is through these transformations that occur in the hypothalamus, which prevent us from making distinctions between women's physical and emotional issues and where they become synonymous.

The Unpredictable Pituitary Gland

Through the pituitary gland and its extensive connection to the nervous system, hormonal changes due to the stress response and its accompanying alterations in neurotransmitters, can become entangled with the female characteristics and responses of this gland, causing unpredictable changes in women's emotional well-being as well as their hormones. Where the pituitary gland normally depends on stable levels of serotonin to help foster contentment, stability and optimism in women to assist them through their childbearing years, interference from rising cortisol levels can reduce serotonin levels causing sadness, irritability and moodiness during the cycle. Where dopamine usually encourages a healthy assertiveness and determination that supports women in their caring and protective roles, high cortisol levels diminish its levels, causing women to feel less confident and more dependent. Where noradrenalin levels normally help focus the mind and form memories that foster healthy relationships and raise awareness of potential threat or danger, rising cortisol levels can cause noradrenalin levels to rise, making these memories become more obsessive, paranoid and self-destructive during the cycle. Where endorphins released from the pituitary gland are beneficial in easing the pains of reproduction and making it a less difficult experience, disruption of these levels by high cortisol may cause women to suffer much more intense period pains, breast pains, ovulation pain and labor pains. The alterations in neurotransmitters which occur at the pituitary gland can bring an unpredictability to women's lives as their underlying stability is weakened by the interference of stress hormones.

As the chemistry of women begins to respond to their negative life experiences, the pituitary gland forwards changes to its glands and tissues that can cause women to feel an irregularity within their cycle and their hormone responses. When bullying occurs in young girls' lives around the time of puberty, delays in sexual development and a late menarche can occur due to interference with the release of growth hormone from the pituitary gland. When there is fear and uncertainty in young women leaving home for the first time, they may find their periods stop through the inhibition of FSH and LH at the pituitary gland. In the same way, endless stress in a job can halt the surge of LH needed to initiate ovulation, causing fertility problems in some hardworking women. When mothers become overwhelmed by the responsibilities of family, job and finances, they may experience breast pains, irritability and water retention because of alternations in dopamine and prolactin levels coming from the pituitary gland. The stress of an unhappy relationship during pregnancy may cause cortisol levels to reduce FSH and progesterone levels, increasing the risk of miscarriage in early pregnancy. When new mothers with little support become physically and emotionally exhausted, problems with breast feeding can occur when cortisol levels upset prolactin levels. During menopause, the upset of children leaving home can disrupt levels of TSH released from the pituitary gland, becoming a factor in the start of either hyperthyroidism or hypothyroidism. The pituitary gland and its hormones becomes highly susceptible to changes in women's lives and under the pressure of stress and unhappiness, it can become very erratic as it tries to organize changing messages from the hypothalamus and the nervous system, causing an unpredictability in women's well-being.

The Sad Pineal Gland

The pineal gland is a powerfully emotive gland, not only does it receive emotional impulses from the brain, hypothalamus and pituitary gland, but it also perceives emotional pain through the extensive nerve pathway it shares with the eyes. From the impulses generated in the eyes, women's chemistry is open to alteration. When young girls and women face the dark realities of life, those associated with abuse, abandonment, betrayal, rejection and deprivation, not only do cortisol levels rise, impacting hormones, but nerve impulses from the eyes bring changes in neurotransmitters that affect mood. The dominate neurotransmitter in this pathway is serotonin and the pineal gland contains large amounts of serotonin, providing a clue to its importance to this gland. When serotonin levels are raised due to bright sunshine or when women experience that self-affirming sense of well-being when they feel loved, cared for, safe and wanted, it adds an optimistic joy to their lives. Equally, when light diminishes with the shorter days of winter or when women begin to see themselves as unlovable, inadequate and incompetent, serotonin levels are lowered generating the emotion of sadness.

Because serotonin is such an important part of the health of the pineal gland, women that live with sadness in their lives and have lower levels of serotonin, may find themselves more open to irregularities in their cycle, mood and internal clock. Serotonin levels are influenced by the natural fluctuations of estrogen, which make it an important factor in hormonal health. Through women's life cycles, when their estrogen levels are naturally low, just before menstruation every cycle, after child birth and during menopause, there is similarly a drop in serotonin which will affect the hormonal output of the pineal gland. This normally produces slight dips in mood as serotonin is affected, and can alter the sleep pattern in a minor way as levels of melatonin are reduced, but mostly these go unnoticed by women. But for women who have been living with emotional stress in their lives and already have low serotonin levels, this further reduction can cause them to experience these cyclic alterations much more dramatically. This can cause the black depressions, insomnia and irrationality that are features of premenstrual syndrome, postnatal depression and menopause. Low levels of serotonin enable past emotional experiences to more easily resurface, bringing the drama and pain of old wounds back into their lives, even though the cause is long gone. They can become low, angry, paranoid and obsessive, making them fixate on people and situations, and cause them sleepless nights as the pineal gland struggles to maintain its hormone balance. The sadness women perceive in the world around them can prevent the pineal gland from performing its important role in restoring their hormonal rhythms after hormone fluctuations, causing them problems around events that should be happy ones.

The Sensitive Thyroid Gland

The thyroid gland controls the rate of metabolism, maintaining a crucial level of functioning of body processes, and in doing so also sets the pace of women's lives. How well the thyroid gland performs these actions is a good indicator of how much control women will have over their own energy. When women carry into their adult life the emotional stresses of their early years, or when they are consumed by stress, interference from stress hormones can generate imbalance of thyroid hormones, disturbing this critical level of metabolism and causing either the lethargic slowness of hypothyroidism or the uncomfortable agitation of hyperthyroidism. The fact that the thyroid gland is prone to such extreme variations in metabolism arises from its direct link with the adrenal glands, making it highly susceptible to their influences, especially the stress response. An extreme sensitivity arises from the thyroid gland through the intensity of stimulation which is produced when raised thyroid hormones combine with the stress hormones, adrenalin and noradrenalin in women under extreme emotional stress, creating a heightened sense of anxiety, tension and an inability to concentrate, making women feel as if they were under siege from some outside force. The opposite can occur when the use of adrenalin and noradrenalin have failed to meet the needs of women's stressful lives and cortisol is produced in large amounts to slow down metabolism of the thyroid gland. In the short term cortisol manages to do just that, but as stress remains chronic and cortisol continues to be produced, both the thyroid and adrenal hormones can become depleted causing women to feel the extreme fatigue, apathy, depression and lethargy of both hypothyroidism and low adrenal gland function.

This sensitivity of the thyroid gland is strongly influenced by its important role in the development and management of brain neurotransmitters which is supported through its powerful links with the hypothalamus and pituitary gland. Through this link both the thyroid gland and its hormones become susceptible to the nervous responses of women and their life experiences. As young girls grow and develop sexually their thyroid gland provides a mental and physical stability through its control over neurotransmitters. When stress hormones are produced, too early and too often, they not only interfere with thyroid hormones but can also interfere with their emotional stability. This can result in learning difficulties and mood instability, as imbalances in neurotransmitters can decrease focus, attention, concentration and cause great humiliation in education. These issue may go unrecognized in conditions such as attention deficit disorder, dyslexia or hyperactivity and be a cause for some young girls to become overwhelmed by the learning experience and retreat into themselves. As they become older, these hidden imbalances may become more obvious during times of great hormonal activity, when the thyroid gland struggles to keep emotions and neurotransmitters balanced. In teenage girls a low functioning thyroid gland can cause lower serotonin levels, bringing on inhibition and hesitation in their developing personalities, fostering low self-esteem, inferiority and indecision. As these girls mature, imbalances of neurotransmitters coming from the thyroid gland level may lead to a more dramatic uncertainty and volatility as in premenstrual syndrome and insulin resistance. In menopause, women with thyroid irregularities are especially susceptible to instability as they also have to contend with lower estrogen levels, also disrupting the balance of noradrenalin, dopamine and serotonin and which may bring about moments of mania, paranoia, obsession, lethargy and depression. Which ever direction stress hormones shifts the thyroid gland, it has a potential to make women overly sensitive to the world around them and leads to changes in their energy and moods. Thyroid conditions make women vulnerable and can bring feelings of hopelessness, inadequacy and shame as they become easily overwhelmed by not being able to keep pace with the world around them.

The Grieving Thymus Gland
The thymus gland sits under the heart and because of the strong

links between them, can be easily influenced by all the emotions that affect the heart, such as heartbreak, loss, longing and grief. The thymus gland is a highly emotive gland due to the extensive nerve pathway that it shares with the emotional center of the brain in the limbic area. Through this connection, this lympathtic gland, not only clears away the debris of infection, but also handles the debris of emotions and is, therefore, prone to becoming clogged with emotional residue, leading to problems of the heart, breasts and lungs. This powerful relationship can be felt instantly by thinking about an unhappy incident and immediately become aware of the oppressive throbbing sensation in the heart area, leaving you breathless for a second and with a heaviness in the breast area. Woman often hold their hearts while telling their stories, trying to ease the heartbreak they feel inside. However, the thymus gland also has a very intimate relationship with pineal gland, from which its immune tissue develops, increasing the potential of emotional stresses getting translated into illness.

Through these relationships, the thymus gland is highly dependent on the neurotransmitter serotonin for its normal functioning, and which leaves its associate organs (the heart, lungs and breasts) more open to influences from the emotions and the nervous system. When women are happy and content, serotonin levels are normal, their immune system and the thymus gland performs optimally, keeping them healthy. When women are chronically stressed, depressed or have had a severe trauma in their lives, cortisol levels can rise, over-stimulating the thymus gland, sometimes destroying its tissue, reducing its size, and the ability of serotonin to elicit its responses, leaving them more vulnerable to their emotions and the affect they have on their health. Over time, increased levels of cortisol and a dysfunctional thymus gland can cause tissue weakness and breakdown, a reduction in white blood cells, and an increase in inflammatory compounds. This can cause abnormal growths, such as fibroids and endometriosis and allow the spread of cancer. This is the process by which breast and lung cancers can develop after periods of great stress, trauma and grief in women's lives. If I ask women who come in with these types of conditions, what happened in their lives a year or two before they were diagnosed, they usually respond with similar stories of relationship break-downs, caring for sick family members or the loss of a loved ones. Severe heartbreak and grief make women start to struggle with their will to live, changing the chemistry of the thymus gland and leaving them less protected by their immune system and more open to illness.

The Moody Pancreas Gland

The pancreas gland plays a vital role in the survival of the species through its capacity to maintain a continuous source of energy, whether food is available or not. This vital mechanism, called blood sugar, works through a powerful combination of hormones and neurotransmitters that cause the pancreas to be highly responsive to food so it can maintain blood sugar. From the moment food enters the mouth, hormones and neurotransmitters are involved in carrying messages through the brain, hypothalamus and pancreas, making every aspect of eating, not only, a physical experience, but also a highly emotive one. Through this pathway, emotions become entangled with the workings of the panaceas and can influence appetite, digestion, weight and well-being. It is no wonder food issues play such a large part in women's hormonal conditions. In fact, the begin-nings of pancreatic problems can often be seen in young girls around the time of puberty, when great fluctuations in hormones and neurotransmitters can occur alongside stress hormones causing a compulsive attraction to foods that sometimes satisfies emotional needs rather than physical ones. For many it is the start of a lifetime of comfort eating, weight obsessions, food addic-tions, eating disorders and mood swings, as the surge of hormones, a wildly fluctuating blood sugar and fragile emotions mix turbulently in the pancreas.

The emotional instability that can arise from all this activity at the pancreas can affect young girls' self-esteem, leaving them open to irregularities in blood sugar should they experience the stress of rejection, criticism or bullying at this time in their lives when they are building their image of themselves. These damaging emotions can cause the release of stress hormones affecting the pancreas, insulin levels and blood sugar balance. With the release of adrenalin to counteract their unhappiness, young girls and women may find an internal anxiety that they then try to reduce by eating large amounts of carbohydrates in the form of bread, candy, biscuits and cake to provide some sense of comfort and ease in their lives. Although carbohydrates do provide immediate gratification, their fast metabolism causes a rapid rise in blood sugar, which is aided by the release of cortisol. With cortisol comes an increase in the amount of insulin produced, resulting in a rapid uptake into cells, leaving the blood stream seriously depleted. The consequence of this is often hypoglycemia, which can cause women to have a ravenous appetite and overeat, increasing feelings of anxiety, irritability, loss of concentration, fatigue and depression. But this condition can move in the opposite direction, as the overuse of the stress hormone noradrenalin begins to alter the cells ability to take up glucose, resulting in hyperglycemia. In this state, glucose remains in the blood stream, unable to satisfy the cells' messages of hunger, with women becoming increasingly anxious about food, as it increasingly fails to satisfy them. Women begin to have little control over their appetite or moods. As high levels of cortisol cause a lowering of serotonin levels, women may find their moods harder to control, their impulses stronger, and their self-esteem diminishing. This can be the start of compulsive habits that affect, not only their food, but move women into problems with alcohol, drugs and nicotine later in their lives. Women with fluctuating blood sugar levels often learn to live with a rollercoaster of moods and emotions that they can find hard to control.

The Volatile Ovaries

Through the process of reproduction, the ovaries contain powerful links to the brain, nerves and the glands in the brain, carrying, not only the impulses that assist reproduction, but also ones that bring about alterations in mood and perception. The brain's neurotransmitters fluctuate as they follow estrogen and progesterone through the cycle, helping to create the highs and lows women experience each month. With extremely low levels of the galvanizing estrogen during the menstrual phase, the stimulating neurotransmitters, serotonin, dopamine and noradrenalin also diminish. This results in a phase where women are less physically and mentally motivated, a general slowing down that provides them with the time for restoration and recovery from the activity of the cycle. During this quiet time in the cycle, low levels serotonin may make them feel slow and inward, low dopamine levels may cause them to feel less socially orientated and low levels of noradrenalin may cause them to feel less mentally alert and more in need of sleep. As estrogen slowly begins to rise again during the follicular phase, it brings a physical energy, and the rise of neurotransmitters brings a mental vibrancy. As women move into ovulation, there is a big serge of estrogen and progesterone, and high levels of endorphins and dopamine flood their blood stream. This gives the joyful exuberance that leads to being highly social and open to all around them, in particular opening themselves up to the possibilities of mating. After this short ovulation phase, women descend back again into a lowered state as progesterone begins rising during the luteal phase. This, in turn, brings with it a decrease in the activity in the central nervous system and a slowness, as they again begin to turn inwards.

Generally women can move through these phases of their cycle without any hindrance to well-being or to the ability to perform. What causes some women to feel these changes more than others has more to do with emotional stress than with problems in their cycle. Stress hormones interfere with the ovaries, changing hormones and neurotransmitters and enabling emotions to resurface with all their rawness and pain. This is best illustrated in the condition of premenstrual syndrome, where the critical balance between estrogen and progesterone is lost, leaving estrogen dominate during a phase of the cycle when it should remain low, causing physical and emotional upheaval in women. During the luteal phase, higher than normal estrogen levels cause correspondingly higher levels of the stimulating neurotransmitters, which can result in women feeling anxious, unfocused, restless and agitated during this phase in premenstrual syndrome. Correspondingly high serotonin levels can cause long forgotten resentments to resurface in an obsessive and destructive way. With elevated dopamine levels, women can feel edgy, restless, anti-social, and become paranoid about those around them. Abnormally raised noradrenalin levels may make their mind race, lessen the ability to focus and cause impulsiveness. Excessive endorphin levels can bring on dark moods that make them feel nothing is right about their lives. All the pain, resentment, anger and shame they have experienced in their lives can come flooding back during the luteal phase, as the neurotransmitter rises out of control, causing a volatility to emerge. These same feelings can also come up in women during times when hormones are in a flux as after giving birth, with miscarriages, and during menopause. An important issue to consider in ovarian dysfunctions, along with estrogen and progesterone levels is the amount of stress hormones they may be producing.

The Apprehensive Adrenal Glands

The adrenal glands defend the body from physical and emotional danger by producing the stress hormones adrenalin, noradrenalin and cortisol. These stimulating hormones keep women artificially roused to get them through their difficulties, but can also be a sign that there is something in their lives they need to defend themselves from. It is a danger they have learned to live with, and even after the actual danger is long gone from their lives, the memory still survives leaving them with an underlying sense of fear, anticipation and apprehension. Although fear can be thought of as a protective memory, keeping women aware of the danger that surrounds them, it can also become overwhelming as the stress hormones begin to dominant their lives. They have learned to live with a certain amount of agitation and anticipation and their bodies and minds have gotten used to the stimulation of stress hormones. They can become adrenalin junkies, always looking for a fast fix whether that comes from challenges, addictions, or compulsions. They may grow into women obsessed in their actions and thoughts, often brooding over situations and relationships. They may become overly aggressive to combat the underlying sense of fear they feel inside, leading to competitiveness or bullying. As the years go on, their adrenal glands become exhausted by the demands put on them and women lose their help in coping with everyday life stresses. When this happens, fear can take hold of their lives, paralyzing them as they become nervous, apprehensive and unable to cope; everything becomes a potential threat, everyone a potential enemy, and life becomes increasingly exhausting.

When young girls start using stress hormones too early in their lives, they may find themselves more vulnerable to the stresses of their later lives, as the adrenal glands become overburdened and less able to protect them as they age. Stress can easily take over their lives and begin running *them*, instead of them running *it*. During sensitive times in their lives (like leaving home for the first time, working in demanding jobs, becoming mothers, losing loved ones, and becoming carers), they may find they are struggling more than they should. As the neurotransmitters, serotonin, dopamine, noradrenalin and endorphins, become as exhausted and unstable as their hormones, they can become the young women that have nervous breakdowns when they leave home for the first time, the ones who change jobs after each personality conflict, the ones that give up their life to grief, and the ones that collapse after their caring role has ended. Stress becomes the biggest issue of these women's lives and as they become obsessed with how they will manage to cope, they can become anxious, edgy, abrupt and defensive. They can become so overwhelmed by stress they often retreat into themselves, becoming loners, unable to cope with relationships. Some are so driven by the turmoil that they feel inside, they can become perfectionists in an attempt to override the chaos and inadequacy they feel. Adrenal gland function is a good measure of how well women can tolerate their own lives and experiences.

Conclusion

Our second consultation has focused on the emotions and as it has unfolded, my hope is that women have begun to understand how their hormonal conditions may have evolved and just how much a part their emotions have played in this process. By the end of the consultation they are usually relieved that they might have more control over their hormonal condition than they thought. In fact, for many it's the beginning of building a relationship with their condition and instead of labeling themselves with its text book description, they see it as a integral part of themselves and can claim back their personal power over it. This is important, especially today, when there is such a push to find an external source of treatment through drugs, rather than an inward source. Without this internal focus, women are often open to the false hopes of synthetic hormones and the limitations of a purely physical approach, often by someone that does not understand their emotional history. Women are not being guided by their illness and many times miss out on their inner instincts that can help direct their treatment and healing. This takes us to the next step in the healing process: how to help women understand their full intuitive potential so they can use it in their own healing experience. Women's bodies often show them what they need to know, but they are often too far removed from them to be able to read these signs. So in our third consultation, we move into a place where they can reconnect with the signs and intuition of their bodies, in a realm where their female chemistry takes them closer to a spiritual understanding of themselves. It is in the spiritual where women begin to really meet the challenges of their lives and the possible *soul-utions* to their hormonal conditions.

Chapter 3

The Spiritual

Third Consultation

In the first two consultations, we have looked in detail at what makes up the physical and emotional lives of women and the influence they can have on hormones. After absorbing and reflecting on all this, many women are now ready to move deeper into the spiritual realm, a place where they can find the unconscious motivations that have driven their hormonal imbalance. It is within this space women can become more familiar with their underlying feminine nature, recognizing the wounds it has received and the healing it needs. Through the spiritual level, true healing can occur, bringing hormonal balance as women find peace within themselves as they begin to work through their own energy and not the energy of others. At this point in the consultations, the relationship has grown between us, enabling both to be more truthful and trusting, and allowing for insight and wisdom to surface from within. I set the room to provoke movement inwards, with background music of soft bells and hollow drums to stir the energy within. The smell of lavender oil laying heavy in the air helps loosens muscular tension and memories so they can both be released. Between us sits a round cluster of violet-blue hydrangeas, absorbing us in the elusiveness of their color.

The spiritual realm is the least understood and most ignored level of being, yet it exerts an enormous influence on women's health and well-being. The word itself conjures up many different meanings for people, but in the context of this book, the spiritual does not relate to religion (although there is a divine quality in the forces of life). It relates instead to the powerful unconscious thoughts, feelings, intuition and instincts that all women feel, and which are drawn, not so much from, a personal or individual place, but from a wider collective consciousness that is also the source of universal feminine wisdom. It is this accumulated knowledge and experience which has driven women's lives and in particular their reproductive cycles through the ages. Through this spiritual consciousness, women find their connection to the energies and collective memories of the universe and, although they may not intellectually recognize this connection, it makes itself felt in their gut reactions to things, their hunches and their experiences of déjà vu. It is felt walking through a wood of bluebells on a sunny spring day, or viewing a mountain range from its summit, or standing by the ocean just before a storm, or gazing at a spectacularly full harvest moon. In these places and at these times, the barriers between the physical and spiritual worlds suddenly seem to thin, making interaction between them possible. The intellect is quieted, the emotions stilled, and as the other side becomes tangible, women suddenly see their place as a part of the greater natural world. Through the fluctuations of hormones and neurotransmitters that occur in the menstrual cycle, women can feel this spiritual awareness more intensely. Through it they also glimpse parts of their true nature, gathering the knowledge they need to live their lives, the experience to know how to proceed, and the wisdom to know when to change. I have come to believe that many of the conditions that are defined as incurable or hard to treat (such as hormonal conditions), are not incurable because the right drug has not been given, or that a treatment has yet to be found, but because many times the spiritual reservoir has not been tapped in to. The spiritual realm can provide the *soul-utions* to some common hormone conditions and to women's health and well-being. We look to the medical profession to treat our physical body, we have counselors and therapists to help us deal with our emotions, but for many, the spiritual realm is one waiting to be claimed.

Undertanding the Female Cyclic Nature

There is perhaps no better place to begin to understand the spiritual level than in the miraculous processes of reproduction and the menstrual cycle; a continual reminder to women of their close relationship with the natural world around them. Through the fluctuation of hormones in the menstrual cycle, a supple framework is created in women's lives that mirrors the larger cycles of life. Just as every aspect of nature contains activities that occur in a predictable pattern (the sun coming up every morning and setting every evening, the tides moving in and out through the day, the moon waxing and waning through the months, the seasons coming and going through the year), women too, find pace in the timing of their menstrual cycle. For early man, these cycles brought a sense of order, continuity, and an understanding of their place in it, and throughout history, the female cycle was part of this universal knowledge. The moon, in particular, held striking similarities to the menstrual cycle and in the moon's ever changing light they saw the resemblance of women's cyclic rhythms. Both had a cycle lasting on average 29 days, and both were divided into four phases; the moon having a dark phase, a waxing phase, a full phase and its waning phase; and women having corresponding phases of menstruation phase, follicular phase, ovulation phase and luteal phases. They saw within these cycles similar qualities that they could connect with. The darkness of the new moon brought a slowness in energy and mind that enable women to retreat into themselves and gather the knowledge that lies within. As the moon began to wax, their energies moved outward, now having the energy to act on the knowledge gained in the last phase. With the brightness of the full moon, women too radiated out into the world, giving all they had to offer from their wisdom. As the moon receded into its waning, so too do women, as they go down to gather their strength again for another turn of the cycle. There is wisdom and universal understanding to be discovered from the menstrual cycle, and as those before us were aware, women should be reminded of its value and the importance it holds over their health and well-being.

If we look further into the life cycles of women, we see a wider cycle that envelopes them. Through the stages of their development (puberty, reproduction and menopause), women experience the ultimate cycles of nature: birth, death and renewal. Through their cycle, women have within them each month, the capacity to create life at ovulation, the understanding of death from the shedding of their womb at menstruation, and the belief in renewal through the new growth forming within their womb at the start of another cycle. Women are part of the fertility cycles of the earth and beyond, and hold its power and its knowledge within their very cells. They instinctually understand life, know how to handle death, and trust in its continuum. For the cycle is not only about reproduction in women, it encompasses all the intricacies that make up the female nature, the rhythms of their life cycles, the fluctuations of their hormones, the pulsing of their emotions and the altered patterns of their perception. With the rise and fall of hormones and neurotransmitters through each phase of the cycle, women experience alterations in their chemistry that affect them physically, emotionally and spiritually. These fluctuations cause changes in women's physical endurance, mental capabilities, emotional responses, and most especially, in their spiritual awareness. Most women intuitively recognize these subtle changes, but unfortunately, not having the means to understand them, they often disregard their importance to their health and well-being, seeing them as a negative part of their womanhood. With such a large part of their makeup overlooked and ignored, women can struggle to understand their hormones, their bodies and their moods, and most sadly, fail to recognize the power of their spirituality.

During every cycle, women experience changes in their mood, behavior and physical stamina, stemming, not only from alterations in hormones and neurotransmitters, but also from fluctuations in the level of activity of their central nervous system and autonomic nervous system, driven by the changing phases. Through the shifts that occur between these two important systems, women experience changes in their levels of perception, awareness and sensitivity, transforming their spiritual nature at each phase. By looking closely at the menstrual cycle and understanding how women change through the phases, they can be more appreciative of the power of their cycle and become aware of their spiritual nature. Through this, women can begin to value each phase, themselves and their womanhood and begin to see their cycle as a positive experience in their life; one that brings rewards, insights and inspirations, instead of pain, discomfort and instability, and bringing them closer to the *soul-utions* to their hormonal conditions.

Menstrual Phase

In this phase of restoration, women are most open to influences from the spiritual side of their being. With all hormones and neurotransmitters at the lowest point of their cycle, they are physically and mentally slower than in any other phase, causing a reduction in central nervous system stimulation, along with an inhibition of the sympathetic nervous system. Both of these lessen their awareness of the external world around them, causing instead a greater inner awareness, allowing for an opening into their spiritual consciousness. In some women, this phase can be almost trance-like, enabling them to meet themselves at their soul level, where their instincts and insights are strongest, and where their creative energies become more apparent. Women often find their minds flooded with great ideas and inspirations during this phase, as their energy is shifted away from their procreative duties and is now available for their own use, making them feel more selfish and independent during this phase. When women do not appreciate this quiet contemplative time in their cycle, and continue to push on as usual, they may find themselves irritated, distracted and craving to be alone.

Follicular Phase

This is a phase of great activity since all the hormones and neuro-transmitters are active in promoting the new growth of the womb lining and the development of a follicle. Estrogen levels are rising, the activity of the central nervous system is increased and high levels of dopamine, serotonin and endorphins stimulate the brain into activity, all making women more highly stimulated. As noradrenalin begins to slowly rise, it starts to bring women out of their trance-like state of the menstrual phase, and makes them more conscious of the external world around them. They become more sociable and tolerant to those around them, as they begin to see people for who they are, instead of through the lens of their own needs and emotions, as in the menstrual phase. This sociable feeling is deepened by rising levels of serotonin and endorphins, bringing optimism, openness and self-confidence. The dominance of rising estrogen causes the rise of testosterone, bringing a physical and mental stamina which adds to women's great sense of well-being during this phase. All this activity means that women have the energy and self-belief to achieve and accomplish the ideas and inspirations they experienced during the menstrual phase.

Ovulation Phase

The positive feelings and sense of well-being that have been created during the follicular phase are intensified during the extraordinary ovulation phase. During this short, three day phase, women feel a peaceful exuberance, encouraging them to be open and yielding for their procreative duties. They are helped through this by the rising of progesterone and the inhibiting neurotransmitter, gamma-aminobutyric acid (GABA), both of which reduce the activity of the central nervous system, making women calm and relaxed during this phase. With endorphins rising to their highest levels in the cycle, women respond to the world around them with an enormous enthusiasm, contentment and joy, encouraging their potential to mate. High serotonin makes them feel very optimistic about the future, supporting their mating instinct, while rising levels of testosterone cause a peak in their sexual arousal and desire and sets the mood for procreation. Now with all their energy directed outwards, a great surge in noradrenalin occurs, stimulating the sympathetic nervous system, bringing a combination that makes women highly conscious of their external world, yet very aware of their instinctual inner world. This gives them a heightened sense of the natural world around them that they can more fully appreciate. They can now become more attuned to the earth's energies, understanding its patterns, ways and delights, and for this short period of time, see and understand their place in it. They may find themselves taking more walks outdoors; enchanted with the birds, admiring of the trees, enjoying the feeling of the sun, rain, wind and snow. The world is beautiful during this brief phase of ovulation and women are open to, and feel part of its earthy, primal energies.

Luteal Phase

As progesterone rises steadily during this phase, the activity of the central nervous system declines after ovulation, causing a lowering of mood, which is magnified by a sharp decrease in endorphins and a drop in serotonin and dopamine levels. This brings women down from the exuberance of ovulation, and causing an uncomfortable edge in some women. But what makes this phase so distinguishable from the others, is the high level of noradrenalin maintained from ovulation, causing a heightened stimulation of the sympathetic nervous system and generating an unusual self-awareness. This brings women inwards again, but this time, without the high amounts of feel-good neurotransmitters. Instead, low levels of serotonin, dopamine and endorphins can cause some women to feel depressed, tense and hostile. These emotions can get mixed with an agitation, and sometimes an aggression generated by the stimulation of the sympathetic nervous system and the stress hormones, and as they move inwards a strong self-absorption can occur. In some women, this descent can intensify feelings, increase memories, and cause negativity, making women obsessive and paranoid during this phase. This great focus inwards should be a positive one, a time of reflection and internal awareness that enables growth and development from the insights within. But for some women, the descent makes them very uncomfortable, as this heightened awareness only magnifies the hurt and disappointment they feel inside in a phase that will not allow them to stay hidden below.

Women should be able to glide through these phases much more easily than they do. They always seem to be fighting their way through the menstrual and the luteal phases; the two phases where the spiritual realm becomes most visible, and where their unconscious feelings and motivations become more clear. What they are really fighting is their internal world, the part of themselves that they cannot keep down during these phases. This is the part of themselves where their pain is held, the hurt is still raw, and they are unable to conceal their true feelings from themselves. Within these phases women are probably closer to their true nature than they would like to admit. These phases offer women the opportunity to view their wounds, get close to their pain, and most importantly, may find the *soul-utions* to their hormonal conditions. There is enormous power in these phases, the same which is experienced during menopause and after giving birth. When women become frustrated and desperate with these phases they often try to stop them with birth control pills or even sometimes with hysterectomies. Many are then surprised to find that their pain does not necessarily go away, it seems to follows them, although maybe less dramatically. The cycle is women's teacher and healer and through it they can uncover many of the real causes of their hormonal conditions. This takes us back to the endocrine system to see how the spiritual realm affects the glands and changes the chemistry of women's bodies.

The Endocrine System: *Accessing the Spiritual*

It is through the endocrine system that women's spiritual awareness becomes more visible. With the fluctuations of hormones and neurotransmitters in their menstrual cycle, an intricate interplay occurs between the physical hormones and the emotional neurotransmitters, all masterminded by the unconscious spirit of women. It is the spiritual energy of women that is behind their menstrual cycle and their ability to reproduce. Such a powerful experience as reproduction could not occur without some input from a greater life force, the same source that supplies women's spiritual nature. It becomes impossible then, to separate women's hormonal conditions from their spirituality. It is the driving force behind hormonal balance and the stability of neurotransmitters. The way women respond to the external world around them changes their spiritual energy and their will to live, generating changes in the endocrine system that affect them physically, emotionally and spiritually. From this fusion, the wounded spirits of women begin to direct their emotions, creating many of the physical symptoms of hormonal conditions. It is not until women find ways of healing their broken spirits, that they will be able to heal their hormones.

This concept is best explained by looking at the chakras, a system which offers an understanding of the differing energies within the body. From this ancient approach comes the earliest notion of the endocrine system, and the first suggestions of the glands. The belief was that energy from the universe flowed through the body in a circuit of energy centers that are aligned down the middle of the body. At each centre was a mass of concentrated pulsing energy, each with its own intensity, each vibrating at their particular color of the spectrum, and each aligned at a specific site of the body. Today we know that these sites of intense energy of the chakras correspond to the locations of the glands of the endocrine system. The crown chakra, at the top of the scalp, has been associated with the pineal gland; both being seen to have an opening that allows for the light of the universe to enter and direct the spiritual will of individual. The brow chakra, also called the third eye, is where it is thought that the hypothalamus, pituitary gland and the pineal gland all work together in the centre of the brain, creating an awareness that can promote wisdom. The throat chakra, lying within the thyroid gland and near the voice box, gives vocal expression and determination, allowing the will of the individual to be verbalized. The heart chakra, surrounded by the thymus gland, the heart and the lungs, determines the capacity for self-love and the ability for unconditional love. In the middle of the body is the solar plexus chakra, close to the pancreas gland and containing the power and individualism of the ego, from which comes self-confidence and self-esteem. Enclosed within the pelvic cavity is the sacral chakra which is where the energy of life force is contained within the ovaries, providing the source for creativity. At the bottom of the pelvis is the root chakra, the one closest to the earth and providing a strong link to the physical world that brings security and safety. Through the subtle balance of the energy in each chakra, women find their physical health, their emotional stability, and their spiritual awareness. It is also within these chakras that women can see how the wounds of their life experiences have been transformed into their hormonal conditions. There is much to be learned from these chakras and their associated glands, for within them lies the key to understanding the female spiritual nature.

The Spiritual Hypothalamus

The hypothalamus is a crossroads where everything comes

together. It provides an entrance to the physical body through the connections with the lower glands; a bridge that links it to the emotional centre of the limbic brain; and a means of accessing a spiritual dimension through the autonomic nervous system. The hypothalamus becomes a gathering place, where the intellect interacts with emotions and primeval instincts, to create the driving force behind the menstrual cycle and reproduction. In this small gland in the brain, women's life experiences are processed, affecting their feelings, thoughts and motivations, all of which have the power to change their body's chemistry. So at the level of the hypothalamus, period pains are more about what girls feel about becoming women rather than about their diet and the exercise they get. Infertility can be more about an unconscious blocking of women's feminine nature than about their blocked fallopian tubes. The acne of young girls can be more about their underlying need for protection rather than the chocolate they eat. The weight and pain of swollen varicose veins say more about the need of women to feel safe and grounded than about the weight they carry. Through the hypothalamus the spiritual will of women determines their physical and emotional health and well-being.

With its control over all the unconscious activities of the body, the hypothalamus forms a link to the unconscious world of women, from which their spiritual awareness becomes more accessible and apparent through the changing phases of their menstrual cycle. This creates a menstrual cycle that, even though is a chemical process, is guided by the unconscious spiritual control of women. This is where women's underlying feelings, motives and drives can become either self-empowering or self-destructing. The messages and the will of women's spirits are processed through the hypothalamus, moving down and around the pathway of the glands, changing hormones and neurotransmitters, altering women physically and emotionally, mostly without their conscious awareness. That is why women are so unwilling to accept their premenstrual negativity as their own, or the voraciousness of their appetite in insulin resistance as belonging to them, or the edgy defensiveness of their polycystic ovary syndrome as part of themselves, or their despondency in menopause as something they should have. Even through women are distanced from these feelings, they are what command a strong influence on the changes in the endocrine system, the immune system and the nervous system and what brings about imbalances and illnesses, even if that surprises them.

The Wise Pituitary Gland

The pituitary gland converts the instinctual messages from the brain and hypothalamus into practical messages to the glands, through which the spiritual will of women is passed on to the physical body. From the anterior lobe of the pituitary gland, women's unconscious thoughts and feelings are transformed into hormonal messages. Through this process, the feelings and emotions associated with life experiences are translated into hormonal messages that affect not only the pituitary gland, but also its associate glands (the pineal, thyroid, ovaries and adrenal glands), creating serious repercussions for women's physical and spiritual well-being. The posterior lobe of the pituitary gland, on the other hand, is directly connected to the hypothalamus, creating a nerve connection with the limbic brain (the seat of primitive instincts), and from which arise feelings connected to women's maternal instincts and sexuality. What develops from these connections are women's desire for sex, their attraction to the opposite sex, their longing to make a home, and their yearnings to start a family. These are the feelings which are part of the female nature, called 'femininity', and it is at the point of interaction with the pituitary gland that these feelings become vulnerable to women's unconscious reactions to the world around them. It is where women hold their unconscious negative images and responses to their mothers and their fathers, affecting their feelings about sex, motherhood, relationships, and themselves as women. It is these feelings that can give rise to the inability to breast feed, problems with conceiving and giving birth, premenstrual syndrome, postnatal depression, polycystic ovary syndrome and breast cancer.

The pituitary gland and the hypothalamus together, constitute an opening into the higher understanding of women, and help direct their spiritual development and their hormonal health. They have been associated through the generations with the brow charka: the chakra thought to cultivate the opposing traits of intuition and intellect. Through the balance of these two distinct parts of the pituitary gland, women get their spiritual consciousness; the anterior pituitary providing an intelligence that sparks thinking, ideas and mental abilities, existing beside a raw instinctual energy from the posterior pituitary. The merging of these two traits together provides women with their great potential for wisdom. When women's life experiences prevent them from achieving this union, not only do they lose out on wisdom, but they may also find a clashing within their personalities: a fight between masculine and feminine, yin and the yang, good and bad, physical and emotional. It is this conflict from which can spring the forces that generates hormonal imbalances. This is very much apparent in conditions like premenstrual syndrome, polycystic ovary syndrome and insulin resistance, where fluctuations in hormones and neurotransmitters are no longer able to keep the nice girl from becoming the bad girl, the sensible woman from becoming the irrational woman, the graceful lady from becoming the clumsy lady, and the creative person from becoming the angry person. When these two collide instead of mingling, there can be power and drama in women's personalities, causing them continual unhappiness and a constant internal battle that becomes exhausting and stops them reaching their full potential.

The Mystical Pineal Gland

I like to imagine the pineal gland as the top point of a pyramid, rising above all the other glands at the head of the endocrine system, marking the spot where the spiritual energy of the universe enters the body. It was for this same reason it has become symbolic of the crown chakra, the highest one, and the one with the closest links with the spiritual world. It is believed that through its interactions with the pituitary gland and the hypothalamus, the pineal gland enables the opening of the third eye: a place which allows one to drift through the conscious and the unconscious, gathering insight and vision, and to guide the passage to the soul. As we have seen previously, the pineal gland has a strong affinity with the eyes, containing the same nerve fibers and pigment as in the retina, not only enabling sight, but also vision. It is this sense of vision that becomes more obvious during the menstrual and luteal phases of the menstrual cycle and which is one of the greatest rewards of the female nature. From the changing light of the moon, stars and planets, a universal knowledge is conveyed through the pineal gland, one that carries the information relating to the timing and rhythms of life and influences women's hormones, moods and the patterns of their lives.

This relationship has even more impact on women and their hormonal health, as the pineal gland is directly responsible for the initiation and development of the immune system. It is believed that in infancy, light passing through the pineal gland activates the growth and development of the immune system. That makes the pineal gland responsible for, not only, the immune system, but also the rhythms of the menstrual cycle and conducting spiritual light to the soul, all of which give it a powerful role in regulating women's hormonal health. Within the pineal gland there is an interaction between the immune system, the neurotransmitter serotonin and the spirit of women, blending them together and forming the important concept called 'the will to live'. When young girls and women's spirits have been broken, levels of serotonin in the pineal gland are lowered, their rhythms and cycle can become disordered and their immune system can fail to keep them from disease, setting up the framework for hormonal conditions and disease. This unconscious reduction in the 'will to live', can lead to a number of serious, even fatal, illnesses (especially cancers) and can be a factor in chronic fatigue syndrome and Alzheimer's disease. In these disorders there is a depression on, not only the emotional level, but also of the their most basic survival mechanism, which lowers the ability of their immune system to keep order and health. With this can come an energy that can act like an unconscious form of suicide, which can be hard to reverse. When women lose their vision, and their attachment to the spiritual, all that moves them is the force of their emotions, which can cause the breakdown of their physical body. Without the healing of women's wounded spirits, the pineal gland can lose its ability to keep the immune system working for them.

The Expressive Thyroid Gland

The thyroid gland sits in the neck, forming a barrier between the brain and the body, and acting as a buffer between the conflicting energy of the rational mind and the emotions of the heart. Sometimes in women's lives they have had to make hard choices when it comes to their own energy, deciding between giving it up to the care and nurturing of those around them, or using it for their own needs and longings. The clash between what they should do for themselves and the pulls of their hearts can sometimes create an energy disturbance in the thyroid gland, as women struggle, trying to contain their own energy. Some lose sight of the boundary that helps them distinguish between where they end and others begin, becoming over-sensitive, easily hurt and quickly giving up their energy to others. They lose their power and control and may lack the energy to confront life full-force, often taking the stance of victims, blaming everyone else for their own inability to control their energy and their lives. The stress generated from these impossible situations not only weakens the energy of the thyroid gland, but also chronically over-stimulates the sympathetic nervous system, causing more imbalances through the hypothalamus, pituitary gland, and the adrenal glands, causing greater disruption of thyroid hormones and creating anxiety and exhaustion for women. The immune system recognizes this detachment in the energy of women and begins to work in disordered ways, attacking their own tissue as if it were foreign and causing autoimmune illness such as Graves Disease, Hashimoto's Disease and Lupus. Without the ability to manage their own energy, women can become caught up in negative behavior such as addictions, eating disorders and compulsions in a desperate attempt to regain control.

The thyroid gland has long been representative of the throat chakra: the chakra which provides the energy to express oneself freely and the ability to verbalize their needs and desires openly to the world around them. When this is lost, women may lose their power to voice their opinion, and the confidence to express themselves. In social situations they may find themselves restricted by their throat, feeling its tightening grip as their nerves and muscles react to the discomfort they feel with the world around them. Many then find themselves holding back and hiding, limiting their lives, preventing them from moving forward and keeping them bound up in their own insecurities. As their energy becomes blocked within the thyroid gland, preventing the energy flow to the higher chakras in the head, an obstruction occurs which not only stops them from reaching their full potential in life, but also forms congestion within the head area, causing ears, nose, sinus, mouth, gums and throat problems.

The Loving Thymus Gland
The thymus gland sits under the heart and has a nerve connection directly to it, creating an association with the heart chakra, which

is all about giving and receiving unconditional love. From this chakra women learn how to love unconditionally, purely, and without conditions from the ego. For many women this chakra contains energy imbalances, as the way of expressing themselves is often tied up with their strong motivation to be loved. Many young girls' life stories are full of unconscious misunderstandings about how worthy they are of love and how far they have to go to get it. Some find a false self-worth by being useful, being the nice girl and giving to others in the hope of proving their own worthiness, and through others they fill their own emptiness. Some see it in over-achieving; being the best, the smartest, the fastest, the perfectionist, attaining what they feel is unattainable to them. While others find love so out of their reach, they resort to attention seeking behavior; becoming the bad and troubled girl to get the attention they so desire. All these situations take women further away from their own energy and potential, and through the block in energy it generates in the heart chakra, women's love can remain very conditional, never achieving the depth of love they are capable of for themselves and others. All the while, they neglect their own needs, trying to achieve this misguided love, while their self-centered drives move them in the wrong direction. Women are easily pulled down this road because of their deep instinctual and physical motivations when it comes to love. Many of the hormones, like progesterone and oxytocin, along with the changing levels of neurotransmitters, bring women into intensely loving moods, especially during ovulation and in pregnancy, when these loving moods help initiate sex for reproduction and make breast feeding a profoundly intimate and tender experience. All of these help to keep women consumed with the feelings of love, always pushing for it, desiring it and fighting for it, even to their own detriment. In the craze of pursuing love, women can often block access to their heart chakra and lose out on the most profound love of all: self-love.

The close association between the thymus gland and the heart creates a powerful relationship between women's immune system and the capacity for unconditional love. When women fail to meet their own needs, the organs surrounding the heart chakra, the lungs, breast, heart and upper arms and shoulders, are especially at risk of illness, as the muscles and nerves supplying these areas are strongly connected to the immune system. The strong sense of control that women use to gain the love they desire creates tension, stress and congestion in these areas, often exhausting them. Without this love, tumors and endometriosis may grow near the hearts and lungs of those not able to love themselves enough and aggressive inflammatory breast cancer can eat away at the flesh of those that have never experienced unconditional love in any form. The arms and shoulders of women with fibromyaglia can ache with unbearable pain as they reach for love that seems unattainable. Women's ability to love, be loved and love themselves unconditionally will influence how well their immune system works for them.

The Centering Pancreas Gland

The pancreas gland lies near women's center of gravity, helping them balance the load of their lives. The solar plexus, located centrally, is positioned between the upper more transcendent chakras, and the lower, earthy chakras, bringing a powerful balance between these energies. This keeps women stable and centered in life, just as the insulin produced in the pancreas gland keeps their blood sugar levels even and steady. If within the life stories of young women there is loss of their personal control to someone abusive, controlling, manipulating, critical or needy, the energy within the solar plexus loses the capacity to build a strong self-esteem, while the pancreas gland itself loses control of its insulin production. Both of these lessen women's ability to focus within, to know what they want and how to get it, reducing their personal power. They may become overly attracted to the power of others, as in them they see what they themselves lack. Because these relationships are held together by a negative attachment, in time, women can become consumed and exhausted by these same things they are attracted to. Their lives can become chaotic as they are not working through their own energies, but through those of others. They may find themselves riddled with insecurities, indecision, moodiness and unhappiness that they are desperate to change. They may look to comfort themselves in acts of immediate gratification, whether that has to do with food, alcohol, clothes, jewelry and men, anything that will, in the short term, satisfy their inner spiritual emptiness.

When energy in the pancreas is not balanced, women can become full of extremes and everything they do has drama to it; they are either exuberant or depressed, lonely or gregarious, hungry or stuffed, obese or thin; there is no in-between for them. In many ways, this turbulence is similar to that contained in their blood sugar, raising wildly and crashing violently, as they try to feed a needy appetite. Ups and downs drag them through life, exhausting them and always keeping them looking for the next high. They can become hyper and easily distracted, never really finishing what they start and never really believing in what they are doing. They may have no control over their appetites, their bodies or their lives, and their insecurities and depression can drive them to addictions and eating disorders. With the pancreas gland's close proximity and nerve connections to the digestive organs, women's personal lack of fulfillment can cause indigestion, their worries the start of peptic ulcers, their low self-esteem brings on bulimia, their lack of control leading to anorexia, their anger turning to gallstones, their resentments encouraging bowel cancer, and their anxiety bringing on hot flushes. Without the pancreas bringing order through the chakras, women can spiral out of control, lacking the spiritual connection to bring their lives together.

The Creative Ovaries

Every month, through activities within the ovaries, women get the opportunity to create life; a process that carries with it a great potential for creative energy. When conception does not occur through ovulation, the energy generated by this process does not just disappear, but becomes available to women during their luteal phase. However, in this phase, creative energy transforms into a vitality and drive that can become conflicting when progesterone dominates and its instinctual feminine attributes rise, sometimes making for a confused awareness. This is when the increase in inhibiting neurotransmitters can cause emotions to rise to the surface; where an intense arousal can emerge through the activation of the sympathetic nervous system, and where women begin to fixate on their internal world. The accumulation of all these developments generates a frenzy of activity, pulling the body and mind with a centrifugal force that creates the wild energy of creativity. So although every cycle does not end in conception, women will, nevertheless, be empowered with a creative energy during the luteal phase that is fuelled by a sexual energy, a sharp awareness and a deep instinctual drive, bringing passion and inspiration into their lives. Unfortunately, in some women, this wild energy can get misinterpreted when they move inwards, finding pain instead of inspiration and bringing destruction rather than creativity. It really is a time when women could create some of their best works, whether that happens to be through their jobs, art, families, homes or in redesigning their lives. Women keep trying to live as they normally do during the luteal phase, even though they have a wild energy looking for a creative outlet; its no wonder this phase is associated with so many problems.

The ovarian energy of creativity is closely associated with that of sexuality. I can often feel a wild rumbling energy over the ovaries of many of my patients; a grappling in the ovaries between two opposing life forces: the calm, yielding power of progesterone and the dynamic and dangerous sexual power of estrogen and testosterone, creating a polarity within the ovaries between feminine and masculine energies. Through their cycle, women are continually pulled between these energies and when there is an unconscious discomfort with their female or male role models, there can be a clash of energy which can create problems involving sexuality and reproduction. Their mother may have been lost to drugs or alcohol, to many lovers, or to the depression of a lost and nostalgic dream. Their father may have been distracted and distant, frightening and impossible to please, or just a lingering angry memory. With each turn of the cycle, and a change in the dominance of these opposing hormonal energies, disturbing feelings and conflicts can arise from the ovaries, becoming some women's lifetime struggle with what is expected of them as women, partners, daughters and mothers. They hold these wounds within the ovaries, a place representing the sacral chakra, hindering them from growing into self-confident, assured, sexually healthy women. Restriction of sacral energy can block sexual development on all levels and can become so powerful that it can generate disorders that are instinctively protective to their sexuality. Women may experience conditions which unconsciously block entry to their sex organs like vaginitis, cervical disease, cystitis and thrush; some may find conception hampered by conditions such as polycystic ovary syndrome and endometriosis; others find their lives so compromised by fibroids, heavy bleeding and migraines that it helps to justify their inability to move forward in life. When the energy in the sacral chakra has been exhausted by the demands of being suppressed, bowel, endometrial or ovarian cancers are capable of progressing. No matter what age women are, the energy from the ovaries needs an outlet to help sustain their health and well-being.

The Security of the Adrenal Glands

Infants' needs are few, but essential to their survival; needing to feel safe, warm, fed and nurtured, all of which lead to an attachment to those in charge of their care. Forming these bonds early in life gives them a feeling of security, enables them to build healthy relationships and gives them a strong sense of belonging, all essential to their development into healthy adults. When very young children fail to make these necessary bonds, whether through neglect, adoption, separation or death of parents, they lose the vital ingredient that binds them to the world around them and enables them to be well-balanced and grounded in the world that surrounds them. It is the adaptive nature of the adrenal glands that takes over in these cases, where the family has failed. Deprived of this external security, they become dependent on the internal security that comes through the output of stress hormones, providing a chemical support that helps them through their early deprivations, but also keeps them in a self-protective mode which can dominate their lives. They can become women that need to control their surroundings in an effort to feel secure, and may become inflexible, retentive and compulsive to meet this great need. As grown women they can become fearful to leave the confines of their dysfunctional families, or may choose to stay in abusive relationships, preferring the safety they offer rather than being alone, no matter how detrimental they are to them. These are the same women that confuse outsiders by how much exploitation they are willing to accept in relationships; for no one can understand the basic needs that are getting met through these relationships and sometimes even they forget.

This great need to feel safe can make women live in extreme situations, look foolish, manipulative or weak, as they do whatever it takes to make them feel secure. The motivating force behind their drive comes from their root chakra, a chakra often associated with the adrenal glands and involving the deepest instinct to survive. Denied the ability to move this energy upwards into the higher chakras, this energy becomes heavy and overbearing in their lower body, putting pressure on the pelvis, hips, legs and feet, causing problems due to the stress and strain of this energy. Their womb may cramp with period pains, their bowel tensed tightly with irritable bowel syndrome, their lower back in clenching spasm, or their sciatic nerve compressed with pain. Similarly, their hips and knees may become swollen from the weight of inflammation, their varicose veins distend from this pressure, their bones become weary with osteoporosis, their blood weaken with anemia, and their feet become infected with athletes foot, as the energy of the root chakra is blocked from moving beyond the confines of the lower body. Women are left living with an internal chemistry and energy that is dominated and directed by their feelings of self-preservation and are always looking for ways to feel rooted and connected, whether they are good or bad ways.

Conclusion

The realities of women's procreative abilities is that they are left with a profound spiritual awareness and energy linked to the life force of the universe. Through this spiritual consciousness, hormonal conditions become connected to the spiritual will of women. So when life experiences break the spirit of women, it inevitability affects their life force, having an immense influence on their reproductive capacities and their hormonal balance. We cannot separate hormonal conditions from the inner workings of women, nor can we treat them with external, synthetic, inorganic materials like hormone replacement therapy, birth control pills or antidepressants. In hormonal conditions we are working with something much more powerful; we are working with the soul of women and treatment must enable women to meet their souls in order to heal their wounds. But maybe this is also what scares women so much when it comes to hormones. Hormones make more obvious all they are trying to hide and they will never let women rest until they have taken care of business. Even through menopause, hormones will keep women uncomfortable in the hope of provoking change, for the spirit of women is always striving for wholeness. By now I hope it is clear that we cannot change the physical body, or calm emotions, while the spiritual wounds are running the lives of women. For spiritual healing to occur, women must find ways of meeting their wounds again, so they can change their perceptions of them and work with them at the level of their origin. Through their spiritual awareness, women find the *soul-utions* to their hormonal conditions, all of which will become more obvious in the next chapter where the activities that allow for healing to occur are explored.

Chapter 4

Healing Ways: *The Soul-utions*

Later Consultations

Having now reached a point in consultations where the source of women's spiritual wounds have become more obvious, they are now in a position to be able to begin the healing process. Many times in the earlier consultations, there may have been diet advise given to help curb moods, herbs to reduce discomfort, or hands-on-healing to help soothe the emotions, but mostly healing comes after the depth and extent of the wounds have been established. During these healing consultations, the room plays a vital role, and by now may have become a sanctuary for women; a place where they can feel safe, comforted and at ease. As soon as they open the door, the smell, sounds, and peace within the room helps to turn their attention inwards, enabling them to leave behind the children, dogs, appointments and shopping, and focus their awareness on themselves and the process of healing. The burning of oils of bergamot and lemon fill the room with an absorbing scent that halts the activity of their minds and elicits a spontaneous, pleasant sensation while bringing a cleansing atmosphere into the room. As they sit down their eyes wonder to the dried grasses sitting in a vase against the open window. As the sun pours in on them, it casts their silhouettes, and with a slight breeze their shadows begin to dance against the walls, bringing a dreamy movement into the room.

Just as illness occurs at different levels, so too does healing. I think every woman's experience of healing is different, will occur at different stages in their lives and may mean different things to different women. Healing is about changing the conscious and unconscious negative motivations and beliefs that work against women's true nature. It's about learning what is right for them and believing and trusting in their instincts and intuitions. Healing means living unconditionally, giving up expectations and living freely and lovingly from the soul. With this comes a balancing and restoring, bringing women's physical, emotional and spiritual aspects in line with one another, and all working with the same positive intention: to bring health and well-being. True healing is rarely achieved at one go, but usually occurs through small incremental steps, each one helping to make women more intimate with themselves, and each bringing them closer to understanding themselves.

The early activities that initial healing may seem mundane and simplistic, but are actually the building blocks that help to achieve self-love. The start of healing, for some women, may mean changing the way they eat their breakfast, and instead of rushing it with a breakfast bar and coffee on their way to work, they wake up earlier and prepare a bowl of fresh fruit, oats, yogurt, and a cup of herbal tea, letting their body know they care enough to give it the time and food it desires. Others may find it healing to say positive affirmations throughout the day, to offset the unconscious self-ridicule that has become so habitual that they can no longer hear themselves. In some, it may mean making the decision to find a therapist to help them work through the wounds and the patterns that keep holding them back in life. Others may find studying a discipline, like mediation, helpful in focusing their mind and getting closer to their own energy. For some women it may be learning to express themselves through crafts, art or through education, to help connect with their innate potential.

All of these activities bring healing to women on some level, bringing them closer to knowing who they really are and what their needs are. They reinforce their self-importance and enable them to develop a relationship with themselves which fosters inner happiness and peace. More importantly, these activities send the right kind of messages to all the cells in their bodies, letting them know they care about staying healthy. In turn, the cells start working for women, the glands work more in sync with each other, the hormones become more balanced and the neuro-transmitters more stable, all bringing a sense of health and well-being. It does not matter how women starts their healing journey, all they need to do is begin it. Once they feel its rewards, they will never want to go back, and will continue to take more steps in the right direction. Women may even notice the path becomes easier for them as sign posts begin to appear, guiding them along their journey. In healing, positive energy follows positive intention, and women do not have to worry if they are doing the right things, they will be able to feel it.

Healing Through the Endocrine System

The Parasympathetic Nervous System

To understand how healing methods can change the health and well-being of women we have to bring our focus again to the endocrine system, where, not only do we find the origins of hormonal illnesses, but also the potential to heal them. Through the hypothalamus, we have mainly got to know the autonomic nervous system through one of its branches, the sympathetic nervous system and the stress hormones it produces. But there is another branch of the autonomic nervous system, a kind of alter ego to the sympathetic nervous system, called the parasympa-thetic nervous system, which is vital to the understanding of the healing process. Within the contrasting nature of these two systems is found the *soul-utions* to hormonal health for women. While the sympathetic nervous system works to stimulate in emergencies, burns energy, excites muscles and brain function, breaks down tissues and causes deterioration through its processes; the parasympathetic nervous system slows everything down, relaxes muscles, reduces brain activity, makes energy, restores strength, rebuilds tissues and brings healing and comfort. Where the sympathetic nervous system can cause digestion upsets like irritable bowel syndrome, indigestion, acid reflux and insulin resistance; the parasympathetic nervous system improves bowel function, calms a nervous gut, balances blood sugar levels, and improves liver function. Over time, the sympathetic nervous system can exhaust the adrenal glands and can over-stimulate the thyroid gland; while the parasympathetic nervous system restores balance back to all of the glands. The sympathetic nervous system is activated by the emotions of fear, rage, anger and pain; while the parasympathetic nervous system is activated by relaxation, soft music, a gentle touch or a loving thought. Instead of using the stress hormones, adrenalin, noradrenalin and cortisol in a defensive and aggressive way, as the sympathetic nervous system does; the parasympathetic nervous system uses endorphins, GABA and serotonin, all neuro-transmitters that bring a relaxing, joyful calm that enables coping in a more rational and peaceful manner.

The extraordinary ability of these two distinct, yet compatible, parts of the autonomic nervous system means that in times of stress, the body can be pushed hard by the sympathetic nervous system to get the individual through their traumas and tribula-tions, because it also has the capacity to replenish and restore afterwards what has been used up through the parasympathetic nervous system. But unfortunately, the time and capacity for restoration is not something that is given time or priority in western culture. So many women continue to push themselves, even after their threats are gone without thought to the detriment of their bodies and mind. This is especially damaging to women who have had difficult early life experiences where they have learned to depend on the workings of their sympathetic nervous system for support. Their bodies slowly get used to the stimu-lation of stress hormones getting them through their days, and without realizing it, many women become hooked on this heightened state of arousal, relying on stress hormones to keep their exhausted bodies and minds performing. This agitated arousal becomes a part of some women's normal existence, bringing an edginess to their nature, and causing some to overachieve, some to underachieve and some to remain griped by the fear and anxiety of stress hormones. It is having to cope with this underlying discomfort that pushes many women to rely on negative coping strategies, like drinking, drugs, eating, gambling, sex, road rage and shopping, to help release the enormous amount of stress building up within them, as they are pushed, more and more, towards sympathetic nervous system domination. These activities only keep women more agitated, throwing more stress hormones into the blood stream, producing more stimulating neurotransmitters, with more uncomfortable feelings and health consequences. The more women are pushed in this direction, the further away they move from the comforting workings of the parasympathetic nervous system and may become more prone to the exhaustive and degenerative state of an overused stress response.

The only real way to save women from the domination of the sympathetic nervous system is for them to learn ways of encouraging the parasympathetic nervous system. The types of activities that help stimulate this are things like breathing exercises, mediation, positive affirmations, prayer, reflexology, massage, visualization, hypnosis, or being in a peaceful and beautiful setting. These produce the same sensation as experienced while rocking in a hammock or swaying in a swing, having your hair stroked, or talking to someone who says nice things to you. These actions start a gentle wave of serenity that passes down through the whole body, bringing a soothing calm that quiets the mind and relaxes the body, freeing women from tension, stress and worry and achieving what is known as 'well-being'. It is in this state that healing can occur with the restoring of tissues, the balancing of hormones and the encouragement of positive energy. In the parasympathetic mode women's activities and habitual behaviors are slowed just enough to enable them to bring the polarities of their nature back into sync. It realigns the relationship between their physical, emotional and spiritual worlds, and the intellectual and intuitive aspects of their consciousness, bringing them into an equilibrium that allows a mutually beneficial exchange of healing energy. This is the process through which wholeness is restored and healing is actualized. In this chapter we will explore the various healing tools used to achieve healing, and bring optimism and well-being back into life.

Nutritional Healing

The way women feed themselves is a profound statement about how they feel about themselves physically, emotionally and spiritually. There is no other regular activity that carries such a powerful potential to either heal or harm them. The time and effort women put into their food is a good indicator of how they care for their physical body; the types of food they eat reveal the state of their emotions; and the amount of food they eat can show how disconnected they are from their spirit; all making nutrition a good place to start the healing process. Nutrition has an affect on the autonomic nervous system, and women's food choices can play a role in determining which branch of it they will use more regularly. Foods that are nourishing and alkaline, like fruits and vegetables, will help keep the parasympathetic nervous system more dominate, promoting efficient digestion and bringing an inner contentment. Those foods that are low in nutrients, high in sugar, full of salt and preservatives, over-stimulate the body, causing acidity and stimulating the sympathetic nervous system, causing anxiety, irritability and digestive problems. Just think about how it felt after your last binge on that big bag of potato chips, that extra large chocolate bar, or that quart of chocolate ice cream. Usually, after the immediate rush of excitement, what follows is an uncomfortable fullness, along with an uneasy agitation, that is followed by guilt, remorse, self-loathing and depression. For the sake of the immediate gratification of food, women can negatively affect themselves physically, emotionally, and spiritually and achieve nothing positive in return. But if you think about what is felt after eating a colorful fresh salad, a bowl of home-made vegetable soup, or a cool glass of freshly pressed carrot, ginger and apple juice, the sensation is very different. They can feel enlivened by the pulsing energy of the food, pleased with themselves that they have taken the time to prepare it, and at peace with themselves for the wholesome nourishment which feeds them on all levels. Food works in powerful ways and women should remain aware of how food can affect them at all levels of their being, as we will delve in to now.

Physical Aspects of Nutrition

Today, in the extremes of the fast-food and gourmet food cultures, women often forget the essential purpose of food, which is to keep them healthy and active. Through the digestion of food they should get all the carbohydrates, proteins, fats, vitamins and minerals they need to make the energy to perform, the nutrients to sustain tissues and the building blocks to make hormones and neurotransmitters. The type of foods women eat influence how well their glands function, the balance of their hormones, the regularity of their cycle and the health of their reproductive tissues. For each gland to maintain a full and sustaining metabolism it cannot do without all the appropriate amounts of the B vitamins, magnesium and protein from the diet. Hormonal balance can be affected if the diet of women does not supply enough of the amino acid, tryptophan, to make serotonin and melatonin in the pineal gland, sufficient iodine to makes thyroid hormones in the thyroid gland and enough zinc to help the thymus gland perform its immune activities. The menstrual cycle can be interrupted by the inadequate amount of Vitamin A, proteins and zinc that facilitate the hormone release of FSH and LH from the pituitary gland and the subsequent production of estrogen and progesterone at the ovaries. Without sufficient Vitamin E, essential fatty acids, protein or iron, women would not be able to maintain the cyclic growth and development of the womb lining or the health of their breasts. All of these nutrients must be supplied through the food supply in order to maintain a women's reproductive health.

Emotional Aspects of Nutrition

The choice of foods women eat can either have a stabilizing affect on their emotions, or be the cause of bouts of uncontrollable irritability and moodiness. Fresh fruits and vegetables supply women with vitamin C, which feeds the adrenal glands, helping them to improve their ability to cope with stress, making their lives easier and more manageable. Eating fast-foods that are depleted of vitamin C will place a burden on the adrenal glands, reducing women's tolerance to life stresses. The mineral, magnesium, found abundantly in green vegetables, is vital to the emotional health of women, and when their diet is deficit of this major mineral, it can be the cause of muscle tension, anxiety, palpitations, fatigue and depression during the cycle. The B-vitamins found in grains support metabolism and the nerves, keeping women more relaxed and steady through the day, but can be easily depleted by alcohol, coffee, sugar and fast-foods, causing more tension, irritability and depression. The levels of omega 3 essential fatty acids found in fish and seeds, can improve brain function and keep women lively, active and focused, but their benefits are being rapidly marginalized by the ever-growing presence of omega 6 oils, contained in processed and fast foods. The chromium found in nuts has the ability to deliver a more balanced blood sugar and foster emotional stability, but with a food supply which excessively promotes processed sugar, blood sugar instability is becoming more of an issue to hormones and health. The fast release of sugar into the blood stream upsets blood sugar balance causing, in some women an adrenalin rush bringing on anxiety, agitation, palpitations, restlessness and loss of concentration within minutes. It is often a trigger in premenstrual rages, afternoon fatigue, insomnia and migraines, and one of the most damaging foods to hormonal balance. While initially being comforting, some foods can only bring women further down into a spiral of self-destruction, often serving as a reminder of their inadequacies and vulnerabilities. The wrong food can bring out the worse in women, and dramatize their weaknesses, making them cry, rage, scream and retreat.

Spiritual Aspects of Nutrition

With control and self-discipline in food choices, women can cultivate their spiritual consciousness, building their confidence and positive self-image. Feeding oneself is the ultimate action of self-love, and eating good food creates good vibes and good intentions all around. There are reasons why fasting has been an integral part of many different religions and fruits are laid at alters as offerings. With the abundance of foods today, we are forgetting that there is something sacred about food; live, healthy food carries the energy of life, an energy that vibrates with life force. When digested, healthy food has the power to increase positive energy, bringing balance, focus, awareness and wisdom. The foods that tend to hold this energy are those that are fresh and raw, especially fruits and vegetables, in addition to sprouts, seeds, nuts, seaweeds and wild foods. These are full of live energy, enzymes and nutrients that have a positive reaction when ingested and are life-affirming. They give women their stamina, hope and optimism in life, and keep their spirits alive, enabling them to live up to their true potential. Foods that deplete energy and life force are those that have had their nutrients processed out, and are essentially dead foods, such as junk foods, sweet drinks, bakery products, candy, sugar and alcohol. Starved of life force, they become acidic and unhealthy to the body, causing disease and bringing the spirit down with confusion, negativity and emptiness. Food is about maintaining life, and when women's food choices are healthy ones they are sending an important message to their cells, one that says they are worthy and want to remain healthy.

Don't disregard food in healing, it has enormous therapeutic possibilities. When everything else is going wrong in life, good food can be the difference between health and illness. Although some women may be having a stressful time in their jobs, eating sensibility could get them through the day much easier. Even though they have been told they have gallstones, staying away from fatty foods could keep them from having their gallbladder removed. When they have had another of those premenstrual rages that are jeopardizing their relationships, reducing sugar could help keep their mates. Their skin has flared up with itchy spots, they know its time to avoid bread, chocolate and sugar in their diet. When they wonder why they have become so sluggish and tired in the afternoons, they should think about what they ate for lunch. Food is a power tool for women, it can give them back control over things they may have felt they have little control over, and be the start to their overall empowerment.

Control over food is becoming even more of an issue today, as women are facing more hazards from their food than ever before. There are estrogens and growth hormones coming through the food chain from meats, poultry, dairy, plastics and packaging; fish and seafood can often be contaminated with toxins and heavy metals, and vegetables and fruits bombarded with pesticides, all interfering with the workings of the endocrine system. For many busy working women, the ease of ready prepared foods is too attractive to pass up, many buying two to three of their meals from a shop. These foods not only introduce additives, flavorings, sugar, salt and soy to their daily diet, but also cut out the beneficial feelings that come from preparing food yourself. As people become more distanced from the preparation of their own food, they lose out on the energy and love that can go into it when prepared with care. The energy put into food preparation is something not measured or thought of as nourishing, but is a powerful and necessary aspect to healthy food. Just think back to the last time someone made you a carefully prepared homemade meal and the feelings that came up. Food has an energy that can be enhanced by love, or diminished in the hands of those with no thoughtful intent. The handling of food is as important as the nutrients it contains, and should be used and prepared unconditionally to enhance its energy and potential. The same can be said for the way in which people eat today, instead of it being a ritual that brings people together to reinforce their connections, it now commonly occurs on the run, behind a desk, in front of the television or computer, or alone. The further women remove themselves from their food, the more isolated they become from themselves and the harder it will be to keep themselves healthy and happy.

Herbal Healing

One of the great benefits of using herbal medicine in the treatment of hormonal conditions is that a variety of herbs can be mixed together to form a remedy that is specific to women's symptoms and conditions, while also meeting their emotional and spiritual needs. Particularly with conditions of the endocrine system, with all the various gland involvements, complications of mood and diversity of symptoms, herbal medicine embraces all the complexity of women's hormones. Through a good herbal formula, the physical symptoms of pains, irritation, bloating, hot flushes and heavy bleeding can be reduced considerably, if not successfully alleviated altogether. The mental symptoms of lethargy, confusion and forgetfulness can be improved, fostering more confidence. Mood swings, irritability, anger, anxiety and muscle tension can be greatly soothed, bringing balance back to women. In addition, the underlying vitality and spirit of women can be revived by the restoring qualities that can be found in herbs. Herbal medicine offers the potential to heal at all levels, providing an ideal treatment for hormonal conditions.

But there is something much more compatible between women and herbs that make the two a harmonious healing duo, bringing balance. I see herbs as very feminine in character, containing a vital and active life force that has the power to maintain life, just as women do. They hold within them a chemistry that heals, an energy that empowers, and an intelligence that knows. They can be giving, yielding, aware and resourceful, the same qualities found in the female nature. Herbs can be encompassing in the way they work, bringing together all aspects of their nature, working for the benefit of the whole, as women often do in their female roles. Including herbs in a healing program hastens the healing process, adds power to it and generates a more comprehensive healing. A good herbal remedy will contain a mixture of herbs that heal in a broad and rounded way, creating a sense of well-being. This state of well-being is a vague concept, but one used extensively in the complementary therapies to suggest a state of being comfortable, relaxed and content in oneself so that the individual stimulates their own self-healing. So in using herbs we get not only the power and might of herbs themselves to move the tissues to health, but we also use the underlying spirit of the individual to change the workings of their body, something often missed when people buy herbs over-the-counter. With a combination of these two, a substantial and sustained healing is achieved that addresses the physical symptoms, acknowledges the emotions, and raises the spirit. Herbs provide the ability to work on all these levels at once because, like women, they contain wisdom.

Physical Aspects of Herbal Medicine

On a physical level, herbs bring a positive change to the progression of illness. Through their chemical constituents, herbs alter the function of cells, gently moving them to health by moving circulation, detoxifying, revitalizing and restoring balance. Herbs can be used to stimulate organs to perform better or quiet organs that are working too hard. They can clear up infections and keep the immune system working efficiently. In women's health, herbs are used to relieve many common hormonal symptoms, while also restoring overall hormonal balance. Raspberry leaf tea can relax the tension in the womb and reduce the severity of period pains in young girls. When menstrual bleeding is excessive and causing women exhaustion and limitation in their lives, the common nettle can slow bleeding and restore vitality. Herbs like Jamaican dogwood can relieve the intense pain of endometriosis, while cramp bark can reduce some of the discomfort of fibroids. For women with polycystic ovary syndrome who are having trouble conceiving, chaste tree may be helpful in improving their ability to ovulate. When cystitis returns too regularly in women's lives, a herb like buchu can help clear infections from the bladder. For those with appetites that are beginning to run their lives, herbs that can help balance blood sugar, like cinnamon, may bring some control. When hot flushes and night sweats destroy the hope of a good night sleep during menopause, sage can help cool the body, enabling a more restful night, while providing a source of estrogen at a time when levels are low. Herbs not only relieve the physical symptoms, but can help women gain back a control over their bodies that they thought was lost to their hormones.

Emotional Aspects of Herbal Medicine

If women limit their use of herbs to the physical level, although their symptoms will improve, they may lose out on the extraordinary ability of herbs to soothe and heal the emotions. As many hormonal conditions originate at the emotional level, using herbs that help reduce emotional energy can be the one element of treatment that targets the primary cause of the illness rather than the secondary symptoms. The capacity of herbs to affect emotions comes in many forms, all of which slowly bring back a balance within the personality and brings women closer to their own self-healing possibilities. Herbs can be used to reduce the impact of stress and trauma by providing a stabilizing effect on the neuro-transmitters as St. John's wort does on serotonin levels. Negative thoughts can be quieted and the edge taken off emotional situations with the herb skullcap, a sustaining nerve tonic that make women feel they have more power over themselves. The levels of stress hormones can be reduced by taking gotu kola which helps women cope better with their lives and make them less vulnerable. Some herbs like vervain can reduce anxiety and depression, helping to lessen the dominance of the sympathetic nervous system; while other herbs like rose, can promote the parasympathetic nervous system with the loving comfort and self-confidence it brings. Using relaxing herbs like chamomile can help lessen the unconscious muscular tension that can be the start of many illnesses like irritable bowel syndrome. The anti-depression actions of lavender can lift women from their darkest moments of grief and help them see beyond their pain. When worry takes over the lives of women, herbs that quiet the mind and have a tranquilizing effect like valerian can bring an inner peace back. Used on an emotional level herbs have the extraordinary capacity to assist women through the hard times and lessen the impact stress has on their hormones and their lives.

Spiritual Aspects of Herbal Medicine

While some herbs give women a rest from their physical and emotional pains, others can help to focus them inwards so they can find their direction, peace of mind and become more intimate with themselves. Very often the spiritual wounds and traumas of life keep women detached from their inner wisdom, blocking their intuition and stifling their inspiration. When they cannot benefit from this internal knowledge, they may make the same mistakes over and over again, being unable to move forward in life and feeling their lives have little value. When this occurs, a herb like sacred basil can bring back optimism and balance after the destruction of abuse, criticism, heartbreak and grief; while soothing lime blossoms softens their wounds; and wood betony helps to ground them again. The herb passionflower can quiet their minds and give women the mental space to enable them to gather their energies and thoughts before making major changes. Rosemary can reduce the spiritual tension that keeps their wounds tightly bound within their chakras and allows their energy to flow freely and uninhibited. To help women become friends with themselves again, pulsatilla can help them relax enough to remember the joy that lies deep within their hearts. The power of oats can bring a renewed strength to women that have lost themselves to others. The reassurance and self-confidence that lemon balm can bring restores confidence and self-esteem after coming out of a long difficult battle. The herb mugwort allows for new ideas and inspiration to come forward, bringing clarity and perception to women's lives that their wounds have kept back. Herbs can help women transcend their vulnerabilities, moving them beyond their heavy hold, to find the pleasures that await them when they are whole.

Herbs have a great capacity to heal on all levels, but the mistake most people make when using them is that they expect too much from one herb alone. Then when they do not get the results they were expecting, they become disappointed and conclude that herbs do not work. Herbs do work, and work very well, but in using them, women must be aware of what they are trying to achieve. Especially with hormonal conditions, herbs need to support not just one level of women's being, but all of them for long-lasting results to occur. Women need the chemistry of herbs to restore and revitalize their physical body; they need their ability to soothe the emotional energy powering their hormonal conditions; and they need the support of their spirit to move the immune system into a self-healing mode. When all of these are working together in a herbal remedy, the results are very powerful and true healing is very possible. In Section II we will be looking at ways of bringing the physical, emotional and spiritual energies of herbs together in remedies for the benefit of some of the more common hormonal conditions.

Spiritual Healing

The healing techniques focused on in this section are those which, when done regularly (such as meditation, affirmations, visual-ization and hands-on-healing), can help to achieve a physical relaxation, an emotional ease and a more clarifying awareness, all encouraging spiritual healing in women. They are activities that slow down the sympathetic nervous system while promoting the parasympathetic, bringing a quieting of the mind, relaxing of the body, and a feeling of well-being. As women begin to develop awareness through these healing ways, they begin to see glimmers of themselves as the people they were born to be, and not the people their life experiences have made them. A positive energy is generated with these actions, that washes out the negativity of the past, bringing growth and self-development. They are methods which tap into women's powerful inner resources, helping them find the clarity, intuition and under-standing to change their lives.

The origins of many hormonal conditions, very often, have to do with the loss women feel when their female roles end. Women often come for help, exhausted and empty after their relation-ships end, their children leave home, or their parents have died. The female role is very limited in western culture, and if women are not in one of the prescribed roles of partner, mother, or daughter, they may find themselves lost. These healing techniques can help in revealing other dimensions to women's female nature and help them develop their wholeness and find their possible future roles. Women are very resourceful and adaptive and if given the chance, they can find new possibilities and directions, no matter how hard their lives have been. These healing tools can provide women with the courage, energy, motivation and awareness they need to change their lives and bring hope and new possibilities.

Many women feel the need to change the focus of their lives, but are uncertain how or where to start. One of the big problems they face is how to get beyond the mental muddle their life experiences have created, and reduce the enormous amount of energy it consumes in their lives. Many times this leaves them less time and energy to pursue their own destiny and dreams. Healing techniques provide the starting point to make a first move in the right direction. Whether they are done alone, or with help from a practitioner, healing techniques can be the first step in women's healing journeys, bringing them glimpses of hope, optimism and determination. Once women experience the positive energy that healing brings, they will never want to live without it and it will become the beginning of a new focus in their lives. There is no need to worry what to do next as healing has its own momentum and rhythm, guiding women after their initial step, and carrying the clues that help them know where to go next. You will begin to notice that you are being led by a power from within, a force that takes you in the right direction, and one you intuitively can trust in. Healing brings faith, faith in yourself and in the path your life is taking and, in time, you will begin to see changes in your physical body, emotions and awareness, as your life is transformed.

Physical Aspects of Spiritual Healing

On a physical level, these healing techniques promote the use and dominance of the parasympathetic nervous system, reducing the dependence of stress hormones and reducing the detrimental consequences on health they can bring. These techniques provide the time and the space for tissues and organs to recoup, rebalance and regenerate, bringing cleansing, detoxification and vitality back to weakened and damaged tissues. The yielding energy of the parasympathetic nervous system has a releasing effect on the nerves and muscles that supply the face, mouth, chest, bladder, back and digestive organs. In the short-term women may find that practicing these healing techniques causes an immediate release of tension in their jaw and temples; they may notice less grinding of their teeth at night, their breathing may ease in asthma, their cystitis becomes less frequent, their lower back pain less noticeable and their bowels more regular. In the long-term, these healing practices can bring balance to glands and hormones and increase the immune response, all improving the outcome of hormonal conditions. In time, the chemistry of women's bodies begins to change, and where once they produced defensive chemicals that increased inflammation and wore down tissues, they begin to produce anti-inflammatory and anti-tumor compounds that build, restore and keep disease at bay. These processes can help reduce allergies, infections, fibroids, endometriosis, rheumatoid arthritis, fibromyaglia, candida, the growth of cancers, and balance hormones. There is much to be physically gained from the practice of healing techniques.

Emotional Aspects of Spiritual Healing

Emotions can generate a damaging energy that lay heavy in tissues causing physical and emotional pain. When women are chronically stressed by the lives they lead, or the hurts they carry inside, a tension is created that builds up in their glands and organs, constricting and blocking normal functioning. Within this hold is generated not only their emotional blocks and triggers, but also the beginnings of many of their illnesses and hormonal conditions. The longer these emotions are held at these sites, the more energy they block, the more volatile responses become and the more damage and illness they cause. Through the encouraging actions of the parasympathetic nervous system, women are able to relax enough, mentally and physically, to let go of the hold of their emotions. With the subtle releasing that occurs during healing, negative emotional energy is loosened, shifted and cleared, leaving the tissue space open to the new incoming positive energy that comes through healing. Women often feel a buoyancy after using these healing techniques, as if a clamp has been removed, and they are now free from the heaviness of their emotions and life experiences. Many women find a new spontaneity coming through them, with a child-like energy, tempting them to sing or dance for no reason at all. Healing brings joy back into lives.

Spiritual Aspects of Spiritual Healing

On a spiritual level, these healing methods enable women to get closer to themselves in ways that may not have been possible with the lives they have been leading. Very often they become consumed by their lives, overwhelmed by responsibility, distracted by worry, or desperate from abuse, unable to find the space to stop and think clearly about what they need to do to change their lives. Healing methods provide women with this space, so they can work with their vulnerabilities and see light beyond them. Through the quieting of the mind, a relaxing of the muscles and nerves, and the gentle hold of the parasympathetic nervous system, women begin to focus inwards, sometimes for the first time in their lives. For the brief period of time they are using their healing techniques, they can forget about the children, the mortgage, their jobs and their parents, and experience what it feels like to be with themselves, alone in their bodies and their minds. This centering, where they find their balance, their breath and their truth, is the place they will find the *soul-utions* to their lives. As women continue to practice healing techniques, their lives will begin to feel different, their negativity will not have the same pull, their perceptions of themselves and others will become more positive and they will become less fearful of change. Healing techniques encourage women to move forward in a steady, gentle way, fostering self-respect and self-love along the way. They will develop a deeper understanding of not only who they are, but will also be able to see their place in the world around them more clearly. Their world becomes bigger than themselves, reducing the impact of their personal difficulties, enabling them to achieve a peace of mind and unconditional love that they have been unable to achieve before. With these positive intentions of thought we move on to the healing techniques that will bring women closer to a place in themselves, fostering and guiding them into healing.

Healing Tools

Meditation
Meditation is the act of sitting quietly, anywhere from 20 minutes to an hour each day, the mind emptied of active thought, the body upright and relaxed, and awareness focused on the moment. It takes time to get deep into a true meditative state and often people become so distracted and preoccupied with trying to stop thoughts coming in, that they give up thinking they can meditate. Part of the mediation process is allowing time to let thoughts settle, sometimes taking as much as 15 minutes before the mind is restful. To help with this process, some people focus on counting their breaths, some use the repetition of a mantra, while others find it helpful to visualize a place where they felt peaceful and happy. Once in the mediation zone, they will be glad they persevered, as a heightened awareness settles on them and takes them into a state of bliss. No longer having the weight of the

body, the activity of the mind, or awareness of the ego, they are able to blend into the life force around them. In this state, there is a peaceful tranquility where nothing is important, nothing is pressing and where they can rest, recharge and center themselves. The longer they sit in meditation, the deeper and more profound their experience. Meditation leaves people feeling calm, positive and focused and makes the day ahead easier.

Meditation has been used for thousands of years as a way of connecting to the soul. In the materialistic and secular world of today, mediation is more commonly used by people to reconnect to themselves and to the world around them. For women, meditation can be a start of their journey of self-discovery, helping them to find themselves beyond their prescribed female roles, helping to eliminate the limitations caused by their emotional wounds, and encouraging the self-healing potential of the their bodies. Through meditation the dominance of the parasympathetic nervous system is encouraged and the stresses and strains of life are slowly lessened. If women are able to give themselves twenty to thirty minutes a day in quiet mediation, they will find their lives become easier, the world friendlier and their bodies healthier. With a reduction of the muddle of the mind, women are able to think better, be more efficient and create a space for new ideas and inspirations to come forward. In some women, meditation is the key to their spiritual development, opening up insight, strengthening their intuition and bringing them wisdom. In the little time meditation takes from the day, it brings long-term optimism, clarity and focus, enabling women to let go of the past, stop worrying about the future, and see each day more clearly and rationally, bringing peace of mind and happiness. In the next section of this book we will explore different approaches to mediation, with the hope that one of them will feel comfortable to use or maybe inspire joining a mediation class.

Visualization

Visualization is a healing technique that uses the power of the creative mind to change the way people think. Unlike meditation, where the mind is quieted, visualization uses vivid scenes, colorful images and lively action to bring change to the physical body, the emotions and the spirit. Like meditation, it starts with relaxing the body and centering attention on breathing, but while mediation attempts to quite the mind, visualization actively uses the mind and imagination to find *soul-tions*. With the attention fixed inwards, focus is brought to what needs to be addressed and the imagination takes over, building scenes, reconstructing situations, changing relationships, or manipulating the workings of the body. Through this creative experience, the progression of illness can be altered, negative emotions can be transformed into positive ones, and long-held false self-beliefs can be reversed.

Visualization exploits the power of the mind to change the energy of the body. It can enable women to gain more control over their thoughts, their bodies and their lives by creating the right environment for healing to occur. It brings calm as the parasympathetic nervous system is raised into activity, with the tranquilizing neurotransmitters taking over, causing the muscles to relax, the mind to settle, and body to switch into a healing mode. In this mode, the imagination is used to create positive images to which the body instantly responds with positive physi-ological and psychological changes. When stress and anxiety take hold of women, it can be as simple as taking time out, sitting alone and visualizing themselves in a field full of wild flowers on a warm still summer's day, seeing the colors of the flowers, being aware of the sounds of the birds and feeling the warmth of the sun on their bodies. When negative thoughts keep flooding the mind and destroying the day, women can find creative ways of cleansing them from their minds. For example, visualizing themselves laying in a warm bath full of pink roses cut straight from bush, breathing in their delightful scent while breathing out the negativity that has consumed them. When women are looking for more control over disease, visualization can provide the necessary initial step that stimulates the immune system, like visualizing their fibroid or tumor shrinking before their eyes. Just as women can cause disease through negative thoughts, they can also become the creator of their health by positive imagery, as will be explored in following section.

Inner Child

Through the skill of visualization comes another healing tool that frees women from the wounds of their childhood; a healing therapy referred to as inner child work. The wounds of childhood are some of the deepest, as they occur at an age when children are developing their self-esteem, seeing themselves through the way they are treated by those closest to them. When their self-beliefs arise from bad parenting, dysfunctional relationships, traumas, abuse, grief and deprivations, not only does their self-esteem suffer, but the child is left with a legacy that stifles their emotional development, leaving them emotionally stuck at the age of their wound, no matter how old they grow. They develop into adults who remain influenced by the unmet needs of their inner child. Some become over-achievers to find the validation their inner child longed for, some remain fearful because their inner child was not comforted and made to feel safe, some turning into bullies as their inner child was abused and some staying a defensive adult, always trying to protective their inner child from criticism. They become adults controlled by the negative power of their inner child's emotions towards injustice, violence, criticism, abandonment or shame. They grow up to be adults with emotional triggers, neuroses, addictions, compulsions, anxieties, fears and low self-esteem. While the emotional ties of the inner child are still pulling their strings like a puppet, women can remain lost in their emotional past and find it hard to move forward in life.

When women learn to get close to their inner child, through visualizing themselves at their wounded age, they meet the source of their anger, the origin of their depression, the cause of their failed relationships, the explanation for their exhaustion and the causes of their illnesses. Now equipped with the logic and reason of an adult, they are able, through visualization, to get close to their inner child and experience their emotional pain again, in order to know how to heal. Sometimes, all that is needed is for the pain of childhood to become clarified by adult eyes and healing gets easier. Women are the only ones, at this point in their lives, that can give themselves what that child needed. All expectations of having their needs met from others should be abandoned, as all efforts are usually fruitless and only cause more pain. The hardest part about inner child work is experiencing the pain again, having to recall the extent and depth of their inner child wounds, which are usually so deeply repressed that women are often shocked by their discoveries. But the meeting of the inner child is always an illuminating experience, even if it can be a difficult one. Women should be persistent with inner child work and continue to visit their inner child as many times as it takes to build a loving and trusting relationship with them. Within that relationship is the power to reduce the emotional hold they have on women and the authority to set them both free. From inner child work, women gain back their carefree, spontaneous child-like nature and lose the emotional triggers, sadness and manipulation of their inner child. Most times, inner child work is very successful in making women happier and enabling them to move forward in their lives. There is much to be gained from inner child work for women, the biggest benefit being a child-like joy that returns to their lives, promoted by the, now, healthy child within.

Affirmations

Affirmations are positive statements that, when repeated through the day, help reverse the impact women's negative self-beliefs have on their physical, emotional and spiritual health. Through negative conditioning, such as neglect, abuse, criticism and bullying, young girls accumulate false self-beliefs about themselves that are extremely hard to grow out of, can hold them back, keep them down and be a cause of their hormonal conditions. It is always sad to hear how many women grow up believing they are stupid, ugly or unworthy, when they really are not. The wounds of life often come through as verbal assaults that, when repeated enough, make a young girl begin to believe them. I hear women all the time call themselves derogatory names as they relate their stories. Others will answer their phone calls by saying 'it's only me'. These are profound statements, which are very telling about how women really feel about themselves. The problem with negative affirmations are that they are said without conscious thought. Women often do not realize they are saying them, but each time they do, it confirms to their body, mind and soul that they are not worth caring for. As a result of this, the immune system, nervous system, and endocrine system begin responding accordingly, working under their direction.

A positive affirmation, on the other hand, like 'I believe in myself', said over and over again, until women really begin to believe it, can change not only the way they feel about themselves, but also the messages to the immune system and the rest of the body, improving health and well-being. Positive affirmations reverse the damage of negative conditioning and change the energy of women. They begin to work as soon as they are said and after a few days, women begin to smile more, raise their shoulders higher and begin to feel more positive about life. Some women say they can actually feel a wave of positive energy flowing through them as they say their affirmations. Women are the only ones who know what they really want to hear, so why not say it to themselves, instead of waiting for others to say it and getting disappointed when it does not happen. Women should treat themselves the way they want others to treat them, not the other way around. Young girls may not have had the power or ability to stop their negative conditioning, but as women, they do have the choice to believe it or not. Why live up to others expectations, when you can live up to your own. Positive affirmations provide women with the tools to change how they feel about themselves.

Psychotherapy

Talking to a counselor or psychotherapist enables women to verbalize their pain, so it can be understood and released. Very often, the pain they carry around is a tightly bound bundle of memories, misunderstandings and misfortunes that gets more tangled through the years, causing unhappiness and ill health. It sometimes takes a person with a fresh mind, open attitude, and unbiased opinion to see through another's muddle and help see their way through it. If done in a safe and compassionate environment, in a non-judgmental tone, psychotherapy can be a soothing and enlightening experience. By talking and raising memories, women can become surprised by the volatility of their emotions, the velocity of their tears and then by the calm they feel inside as the emotions are release. Psychotherapy can bring freedom from life experiences that are long gone, but are not forgotten and continue to bring pain and despondency.

So much of women's present day difficulties come through the emotional interpretation of their past and have no real significance to the adult they are today, creating an irrationality from their wound that becomes their emotional triggers. When these are not addressed or understood, they continue to cause repeated problems and oppression in women's lives. Psychotherapists can help rationalize these negative patterns in life and reduce their occurrences, giving women more control over their lives and bring balance, making women healthier, physically, emotionally and spiritually. It can release many years of repressed emotions, reducing physical tension in the body, easing emotional anxiety and helping women move forward in life. It can help them understand why they keep making the same mistakes and why they are able to be hurt in the same way by different people. When women are allowed to tell their stories to the right person, it can offer them not only a release, but also, very importantly, confirmation of their pain, validation of their life, and justification of their existence, something they need to experience before they can let it go.

Hands-on-Healing

The act of hands-on-healing has a long history in many cultures, and is today becoming a popular and acceptable approach to the physical, emotional and spiritual aspects of health and well-being. Healing goes by many names and has many disciplines, but the two most widely used are spiritual healing and Reiki. Both of these healing techniques work with the subtle energy of the universe, the same energy that flows through every person, plant, tree and rock on earth. By placing themselves in a peaceful and unconditionally loving state of mind, healers are able to connect with the higher energy of the universe and disconnect themselves from their own energies. Through their hands, a positive and pure energy can then flow and be used for the benefit of others. This subtle energy flows through the healer and goes where needed, relaxing, soothing, releasing, and bringing comfort. No matter what type of physical, emotional or spiritual problems women may come in with, healing energy will be beneficial at some level. Like the other healing techniques, healing slows the mind and relaxes the body. Unlike psychotherapy, it does not work through the intellect, but from the spiritual level, enabling unconscious thoughts and feelings to be soothed without interference from the mind. With hands-on-healing, physical illnesses can be improved, emotional trauma released and the spirit can be awakened, all bringing clarity, contentment, balance and health to women.

By working through the energies of the chakras, the healer can pick up information about women's life experiences and how it has affected them. As can be seen from the table below, each chakra develops at a different stage in the life cycle and is associated with a specific emotional need, which, if not met, can cause certain spiritual issues in women to dominate their lives. Because each chakra has nerves that branch out into specific areas of the body, it can also provide insight to understanding the progression and origins of their physical conditions. Traumas that occur in early life such as adoption and neglect, where the essential need of infants and youngsters to be cared for has been ignored, can affect the root chakra, causing problems throughout life that can affect the lower body, the blood, bones and nerves. As young girls grow into the sacral age between 5 to 8 years, if they are not protected, they can be damaged by abuse or abandonment, causing them to be more open to reproductive or hormonal conditions. During the solar plexus stage of 8 to 12 years of age, young girls are developing their self-esteem and if they are criticized or made to feel inadequate, their self-worth is destroyed and they may be plagued by digestive complaints in later life. The heart chakra develops during the teenage years of 12 to 15 years of age, when girls are building on their capacity to be loved and love in return, this can often be problematic when they are rejected, betrayed or disappointed by those who should love them, creating a greater potential for problems arising from the lungs, heart and arms. The throat chakra forms around the adolescent years of 15 to 21 years old and provides young women with their voice and determination, which, if stifled by powerful negative influences, can generate problems later that have to do with the thyroid, throat and head area. As women grow into their womanhood they begin to develop their brow chakra, which provides them with the intuition and insight that is their legacy, but can also be their uncertainty if they are not honored or respected, leading to health issues affecting their brain, eyes and nervous system. With the healthy aging of women should come an enlightened understanding of life. This can be inhibited by a bleak despondency that shades the light of the crown chakra during these years, causing illnesses that arise from the brain, like dementia. The list below will help in the understanding of illnesses and their locations in the body.

The healer can intuitively use this chakra information as a way of increasing the healing potential for women. The healer can move blocked energy within these chakras, releasing its hold and improving the workings of the other chakras surrounding them, creating more balance for women. The power of hands-on-healing is that it covers all the issues of health and well-being in one therapy. From the physical level it can reduce pain, increase vitality and slow the progression of illness. From an emotional level it helps relax the body, quiet the mind and allow for emotions to be released, as the hold of the past is lifted. But probably the most significant gift of hands-on-healing comes from the spiritual level, for there is no other method that works so gently in easing women's wounds and freeing them from the pain of their lives. It is always best to work with a healer, but the exercises in the next section are an opportunity to experience your own healing energy, which can be very powerful, soothing and bring positive results.

Chakra	Gland	Positive Attribute	Negative Attribute	Age
Root	Adrenal	Spontaneity	Rigidity	0 - 5 yr
Sacral	Ovary	Resourcefulness	Dependency	5 – 8 yrs
Solar Plexus	Pancreas	Confidence	Inferiority	8 – 12 yrs
Heart	Thymus	Sincerity	Vulnerability	12 – 15 yrs
Throat	Thyroid	Individuality	Submissiveness	15 – 21 yrs
Brow	Hypo/Pit	Insightfulness	Indecision	Adult yrs
Crown	Pineal	Awareness	Hopelessness	Menopause

Illnesses Specific to Each Chakra

Root – Varicose veins, lower back pain, osteoporosis, athletes foot, panic attacks, anemia

Sacral – Menstrual and menopausal problems, premenstrual syndrome, infertility, vaginal infections, fibroids, endometriosis, polycystic ovary syndrome, lower back pain, irritable bowel, cervical, endometrial and ovarian cancer

Solar Plexus – Insulin resistance, diabetes, peptic ulcers, pancreatitis, indigestion, anorexia, bulimia, liver and gall bladder disorders, bowel cancer

Heart – Asthma, allergies, autoimmune diseases, lung cancer, breast cancer, bronchial pneumonia, upper back and shoulder problems, chronic fatigue syndrome, fibromyaglia, glandular fever, eating disorders, heart failure

Throat – Thyroid disorders, sore throat, tonsillitis, sinusitis, teeth and gum problems, swollen glands, deafness, laryngitis, tension headaches, cancer of the throat, cold sores, dyslexia, attention deficient disorder

Brow – Insomnia, brain tumors, stroke, glaucoma, cataract, migraines, nervous breakdown, depression, schizophrenia

Crown – Alzheimer's, Parkinson's, suicidal depression, paralysis, epilepsy, multiple sclerosis

Conclusion

Women hold within them the potential to heal themselves through the food they eat, the herbs they take and the healing they get. These provide them with a holistic approach to their lives that nourishes, restores and heals them on all levels of their being. Just as women can cause themselves to be rundown, ill and depressed, they also hold the power to make themselves feel lifted, well and happy. In a culture where women often give up their responsibility for their health to the medical profession and prescription drugs, it is all too easy for them to lose track of what their hormonal conditions really mean to them and why they are so hard to treat. No one can understand the pain of women, their bodies or their life experiences as well as they can, and no one has the *soul-utions* but them. There is a huge need for women to discover their own healing potential and to recognize the part their life experiences have played in the development of their hormonal conditions. By opening up the current limited ideas about women's health and tapping into women's self-healing ability, women become closer to understanding themselves and trusting in their intuition enough to lead them to their own healing. In Section II, the healing possibilities for women will become more apparent and the healing techniques more accessible as we begin to uncover hormonal conditions individually and see more clearly, the women behind the conditions.

Section II

Common Hormonal Conditions

Candida

The condition of candida is a disturbance in the natural balance of gut organisms affecting the digestive, immune and reproductive systems, and influencing mental and emotional stability. The far-reaching nature of candida's symptoms often causes it to be surrounded by ambiguity, confusion and suspicion, keeping it from being understood, recognized and properly treated. Where most disorders are specific to particular organs and have recognizable symptoms, candida is more like a syndrome, producing many diverse and unrelated symptoms, such as abdominal bloating, diarrhea, constipation, allergies, food intolerances, cystitis, anal itch, rashes, joint pain, headaches, depression, mood disturbances and hormonal symptoms making diagnosis difficult and perplexing at times. Patients rarely come in with a diagnosis of candida, more likely they come in with vague symptoms and discomforts that they cannot make sense of and only through a thorough case history is candida suspected. To further complicate the situation, candida mimics many common conditions, like sinusitis, pruritis, thyroiditis, hepatitis, cholecystitis, pancreatitis, oophoritis, vaginitis and cystitis, often causing problems with diagnosis and treatment. In women's health, candida can often be a hidden factor behind many common hormonal conditions such as fibroids, endometriosis, infertility, insulin resistance, polycystic ovary syndrome, premenstrual syndrome and heavy bleeding without anyone ever suspecting it. I have seen women have hysterectomies, been placed on powerful and expensive fertility treatment, or prescribed birth control pills, hormone replacement therapy, anti-depressants and anti-inflammatory drugs when really what they needed was treatment for candida. These are the same women who return looking for help with their old symptoms after these treatments have failed to provide the results they were looking for.

Physical

Candida is a condition of modern life and has been progressing alongside the ever-increasing dependency on pharmaceutical drugs to treat common illnesses. One of the biggest culprits is antibiotics, with their widespread use to treat everything from the common cold to inflamed toenails in humans, and their intro-duction into the food chain through farmed animals. This has created a situation where the naturally beneficial organisms of the gut are negatively affected, resulting in an alteration in the carefully balanced internal environment of the gut, disrupting digestion, lowering immunity and interfering with hormones. The name candida comes from one of the major gut organism, candida albicans: a normally friendly fungus that lives widely throughout the body. This is one of the major organisms that loses its stability through antibiotics and becomes excessive, aggressive, pathogenic and responsible for many common fungal infections, ranging from mouth and vaginal thrush, cystitis and irritable bowel syndrome to athletes foot. The candida fungus is fed generously by diets high in sugar and yeast, growing out of control and creating many of its damaging and disease-forming symptoms. As it flourishes, it begins producing its own toxins that can destroy the integrity of the selective lining of the digestive tract that normally allows only the smallest food molecules such as amino acids to pass through. The damage now enables undigested proteins to pass through this barrier, causing mal-absorption of foods and these unrecognizable proteins to generate an immune reaction to protect the body from what it perceives as foreign substances. Through this reaction, commonly eaten foods can become immune-active proteins and cause inflammation when eaten, producing some of candida's common symptoms, such as abdominal bloating, wind, pain, diarrhea, constipation, food intolerances, anal itch, skin rashes, skin itch, facial flushing, palpitations and mood disturbances. These symptoms are often referred to as an intestinal dysbiosis, or leaky gut syndrome, both names referring to the mal-absorption of food which occurs. With the immune system now actively involved in digestion, a potential for more problems arises when these immune-active proteins become part of the protein reserves of the body and can be amalgamated into the new growth of tissues in the restoring and repairing process. These tissues now have the potential to be unrecognized by the immune system and become a target of immune attack, producing an autoimmune response (where the body fails to recognize its own tissue), which can be a factor in some cases of rheumatoid arthritis, thyroid disease, fibromyaglia and chronic fatigue syndrome. When these immune-active proteins become part of reproductive tissue, especially the endometrium, which has a rapid turnover of growth each month, endometriosis, fibroids, infertility and reproductive cancers are more likely, making candida an important issue that should be considered in women's health today.

Emotional

The physical burdens of candida are complicated by a disturbing emotional instability that can accompany them when hormones and neurotransmitters are altered by the nature of the condition. As women continue to eat their offending foods, which are usually the most comforting to them, their body reacts in a stress response, with the release of the stress hormones adrenalin and noradrenalin, causing them anxiety, restlessness, confusion and depression after eating. More long-term reactions can occur if candida proliferates in the large intestine, where estrogen and progesterone await excretion in their less active forms. It is in these forms that immune-active proteins can attach to these hormones, making them active again and causing them to re-circulate as immune-active hormones, just as destructive as the immune active food proteins. These produce women that can become overly sensitive to the natural fluctuations in hormones during their cycle as in premenstrual syndrome, or women that respond unusually negatively to birth control pills or hormone replacement therapy. In these women their neurotransmitters are now responding to the volatility of hormones that now have an immune reaction attached to them carrying with them a instability that can feel very unnatural and unsettling. These reactions are almost allergic-like reactions and it often seems that women with candida have become overly sensitive to not only common foods in their lives, but also their own hormones causing them to feel sick, depressed and miserable when their hormones fluctuate in the cycle. These are often the women who begin to hate their cycle for all the pain and unhappiness it brings. The emotional uncomfortability women feel when their immune system reacts with their hormones, could make them feel as if they can no longer handle their own lives any longer. In some ways, this may be true, as the kind of symptoms candida produces, closely resembles adrenal exhaustion, where women's bodies' are no longer able to produce the amount of stress hormones for their excessive emotional needs, leaving them vulnerable not only to the world around them and their hormones, but to opportunistic pathogens like candida.

Spiritual

As a condition of exhaustion, candida makes sense. Many times in candida, women have become so drained by their life experiences they lose their capacity to protect themselves, not only from their external world, but also from their internal environment. They are usually women with low self-esteem who have lost their inner connection to themselves and have been battling their way through life trying to find a way to cope. One of the ways they find can involve giving up power to other people in their exhaustion and allowing them to control their lives. In others, they see the strength and power they believe is lacking in themselves. Their apathy is recognized by the immune system and their ability to protect themselves is lessened as their tissue become more foreign and detached from them. Just as they allowed their lives to be controlled by others, they now unconsciously permit the proliferation of candida organisms through their system. Interestingly, in thrush, their inability to protect themselves is most noticeable at the two major entrances to their external world, their mouths and their vaginas, both becoming covered by a thick white coating, trying to block entry to a world they have become so overwhelmed by. Candida is an opportunistic condition, taking control where wounded women are no longer able to. Much of the dispirit found in women with candida comes from their early years, where blocks in energy, centered around their sacral and solar plexus chakras, leave them insecure and dependent on external influences, whether that comes from those closest to them or antibiotics. Many times, it is the exhaustion from their wounds that cause some women to succumb to antibiotics as they no longer have the strength to look any further. Women with candida need support, encouragement and a belief in themselves so they can gain control back of their lives and bodies.

Nutritional Healing in Candida

Candida's worst symptoms come from eating foods that cause stress to the digestive system. Diet is an important issue in candida and without the awareness of the foods that are triggering problems, candida will continue to cause damage. Unless you can give the gut a period of rest, without the offending foods and the accompanying inflammation, treatment for candida will remain difficult. Keeping a small pocket-sized food diary at hand at all times will help to keep track of any foods that cause reactions and to help avoid them in the future. Because these foods are so individual, a food diary is the only way of helping women to understand their own particular food issues.

Diet Management for Candida
Avoid Yeast
- Avoid yeast products in bread, bakery products, nutritional yeast and yeast spreads
- Be aware of hidden sources of yeast found in many processed foods, which contain MSG, a derivative of yeast found in soup stocks, gravy mixes, tinned soups, sausages, hot dogs, smoked meats, processed snacks such as potato chips, cheese snacks and corn chips
- Avoid shelled nuts, such as pistachios, cashews, brazil nuts and peanuts, which may contain fungus or are seasoned with yeast
- Limit fruits like grapes and dried fruits, which contain natural yeast on their skins
- Check supplements such as B-vitamins and selenium, which can contain yeast

Avoid Sugar
- Avoid all types of sugar, including honey, molasses and maple sugar, artificial sugars and candy
- Be aware of hidden sugars in bakery products, cookies, chocolate, canned foods, salad dressings, ketchup, mustards, processed foods, fruit drinks, juices, supplements, drugs and alcoholic drinks

Avoid Fermented and Mould Containing Foods
- Avoid mushrooms
- Avoid foods that are naturally fermented and contain yeast such as soy sauce, miso, cheese, pickles and vinegar
- Avoid beer and wine

Check Tolerance to the Two Largest and Most Common Proteins in Western Diets
- Grains containing gluten such as wheat, rye, barley, oats

- Dairy products, except yogurt which if tolerated can be beneficial

Supplements for Candida
- Garlic in all forms to reduce fungus
- Probiotics to bring balance back to digestive organisms

Herbal Healing for Candida

A herbal remedy is particularly useful in candida, as you can cover a wide range of physical symptoms, while also treating the underlying cause, which may be emotional or spiritual. Herbs are the ultimate in a holistic treatment when used appropriately. Care must be taken not to interfere with reproductive hormones by the inclusion of hormone-active herbs in these remedies, as they may add to the hormone or immune disturbance as synthetic hormones do. It is also beneficial to go slowly with treatment, as detoxifying too quickly can cause a healing crisis with symptoms more extreme, as the fungus is carried away through the blood stream, bringing all the physical and emotional memories with it. This is one reason women often stop candida treatment early. Care should be used, as many of these women are already physically and emotionally exhausted and need comfort within the remedy. It is highly recommended to work under the guidance of a qualified herbalist for a safe and balanced remedy.

Aims of Herbal Treatment for Candida
Reduce Fungus Throughout Gut
Aloe vera, garlic, galangal, pau d'arco, sweet wormwood, thyme, sage, rosemary, oregano, basil, sacred basil, cinnamon, lavender

Reduce Toxicity and Increase Elimination
Oregon grape root, burdock root, barberry, baikal, dandelion root, artichoke, fringe tree, agrimony, goldenseal

Tone and Heal the Lining of the Gut
Plantain, ground ivy, meadowsweet, agrimony, marshmallow, slippery elm, goldenseal, Oregon grape root, barberry

Increase Immune Response to Toxins of Candida
Echinacea, astragalus, baikal

Improve Blood Sugar
Cinnamon, goats rue, bilberry, gurmar, globe artichoke, fringe tree, dandelion root, burdock root, garlic, sacred basil

Restore and Balance Endocrine System and Reduce Stress
Siberian ginseng, gotu kola, ashwaghanda, licorice, borage, astragalus

Improve Well-being and Help Relax
Skullcap, rose, anemone, valerian, betony, oats, vervain, chamomile, St. John's wort, rosemary, lavender

Examples of Herbal Remedies for Candida

Candida with Digestive Problems (Bloating, Wind, Diarrhea, Constipation

Galangal	15ml	Anti-fungal, Anti-inflammatory
Sweet wormwood	5ml	Anti-fungal, cleanses gut
Agrimony	20ml	Improves digestion of foods
Echinacea	20ml	Anti-fungal, reduces toxicity
Siberian ginseng	20ml	Reduce stress
Betony	20ml	Relaxing nerve tonic
	100ml	

Dose: start with 2.5 ml (1/2 teaspoon) 3 times a day before food, increasing to 5ml when tolerated.

Candida with Skin Irritations (itchy skin, psoriasis, anal itch)

Thyme	15ml	Anti-fungal
Burdock root	5ml	Reduces toxicity

Oregon grape root	10ml	Reduces toxicity
Baikal	25ml	Cleanse, anti-histamine
Gotu kola	20ml	Anti-stress, skin tonic
Chamomile	<u>25ml</u>	Soothes skin irritations
	100ml	

Dose: start with 2.5 ml (½ teaspoon) 3 times a day before food, increasing to 5ml (1 teaspoon) when tolerated.

Candida and Reproductive Disorders (vaginal thrush, endometriosis, fibroids)

Sacred basil	10ml	Blood sugar balancer
Pau d'arco	15ml	Cleansing, anti-fungal
Dandelion root	20ml	Liver tonic, restore balance
Marshmallow root	15ml	Soothing and healing to gut
Astragalus	20ml	Stress, and improve immunity
Skullcap	<u>20ml</u>	Emotional balancer, relaxing
	100ml	

Dose: start with 2.5 ml (1/2 teaspoon) 3 times a day before food, increasing to 5ml (one teaspoon) when tolerated.

Candida with Mood Disorders (depression, anxiety, mood swings, irritability)

Rosemary	20ml	Anti-fungal, anti-depressant
Baikal	20ml	Reduces toxicity, anti-histamine
Fringe tree	15ml	Balances blood sugar
Gurmar	5ml	Reduces the taste for sweets
Ashwaghanda	20ml	Anti-stress, calming
St. John's wort	<u>20ml</u>	Anti-depressant, relaxing tonic
	100ml	

Dose: start with 2.5 ml (one teaspoon) 3 times a day before food, increasing to 5ml when tolerated

Healing Tools for Candida

Aims of Healing
- Find ways of reducing exhaustion and stress
- Gain more control over one's life and physical body
- Increase self-esteem
- Form greater personal boundaries

Meditation for Candida

With candida there is usually an internal, physical weariness and emotional exhaustion that can benefit from sitting in mediation for twenty minutes a day to revive and restore energy. With stress such a big factor in candida, it is good to use meditations that start with relaxing exercises.

This mediation can be very relaxing if done in a recliner chair or lying on a bed or sofa. Make sure you will not be disturbed and the room is quiet. Close your eyes and become aware of your breathing, feeling its regularity and rhythm. Begin to see yourself in front of a still blue green lake in a setting that you feel safe and happy in. It could be a place you have been or one you make up. There is no one else around but you, the sun is warm and there is there is a stillness in the air. Everything feels tranquil in this lovely space. You can see the reflection of the blue sky and the white clouds on the motionless water. As the sun warms you, you decide to go into the water. As you enter, the water feels warm, soft and comforting. You begin to float on your back, feeling your weightlessness as your arms and thighs keep you afloat. Let all the muscles in your body go, as the water takes your weight. You feel light, supported and peaceful. You are floating easily, drifting peacefully, your body feeling like a feather against the water and your mind lost in the tranquility of the setting. With this feeling, allow your mind to drift into a thoughtless, emptiness and be carried away into meditation. Stay with this feeling for twenty to thirty minutes trying to remain in a peaceful mind with your body relaxed and weightless and your mind free and clear of incoming thoughts. If you feel your mind wondering, go back to your floating weightlessness and the comforting surroundings until you are ready to move back into your mindless state. When you feel you have rested enough, open your eyes and continue to rest for a while, taking in the comfort of your relaxed body and the quiet of your mind.

Visualization to Improve the Physical Condition of Candida
Image yourself just coming from a relaxing swim in a calm lake or gentle ocean. You are all alone in this space and there is quiet and peace all around you. You feel safe and happy. The day is warm, but you have begun to feel cool and wet. You lie down on the warm sand and move your body until it fits comfortably into its soft embrace. Close your eyes and feel the sun warm and drying on you. You feel relaxed and comfortable. The air is soft, gentle and dry and you can smell the scent of pine resin from the trees nearby. As you breathe in the resinous scent, it mixes with the drying warmth of the sun, bringing an antiseptic and drying healing down through your body. Feel this resinous dryness passing through your nose, mouth and throat, passing on a cleansing and dryness to the lining of these organs. Begin to image the white, pasty covering that lines them turn pink, clean and fresh. Take a moment to enjoy the healthy feel in your nose, mouth and throat.

Take another deep breath and breathe in the resinous pine oil and the warmth dryness of the sun, bringing it down into your stomach, small intestine and large intestine. See it travel through the miles of intestine, dissolving the sticky white coating that surrounds the hollow walls and leaving moist, pink, healthy tissue. See the weak and open pores of the lining close up and tighten, feeling more toned and healthy. Take time to appreciate the healthy state of your digestive organs.

Another deep breath brings the warm dry air and the pine

essence down into your womb, cleansing the ovaries, fallopian tubes and uterus. Notice how the sticky white coating vanishes immediately, leaving the pelvic cavity fresh, clean and healthy. Take time and experience the comfort in seeing your reproductive organs looking so healthy and fresh.

With another deep breath bring the drying air and antiseptic pine resins into your bladder, reducing the pasty coating and leaving it pink, toned and fresh. Feel confidence that your bladder is healthy and functioning well.

With a last big deep breath, the warm dry air and pine oil are brought down into your vagina, where you can see the pasty white coating disappear from the walls of the vagina. You look around and take in the clean, fresh, pink healthy vagina, feeling assured that you have successfully cleared the candida from your body. Take a moment, feeling the confidence and control you have in your health and wellness.

When you feel you are sufficiently cleansed open your eyes and come back into your space.

Inner Child Work for Candida
This inner child exercise can be done in continuation of the above or on its own.

Alone and in a quiet and peaceful space, give yourself about ten minutes to complete this exercise. Close your eyes and feel your body relax as you take three deep breaths. Envisage yourself on a beach, where you may have been once and felt happy and safe or image your own perfect beach. Feel the warmth of the sand under your feet and the hot sun on your back. You see a large pine tree with a bench under it. You make your way to it and sit. It offers you comfort from the sun and a slight breeze feels good against your skin. You see the gentlest of waves on the waters edge and hear its soft swishing sound. You feel happy and peaceful sitting under this tree. Take a few moments to enjoy your restfulness and the tranquility you feel in yourself.

In the distance a young girl is coming your way. As she nears, she looks very familiar and you begin to recognize yourself as a child. She stands in front of you looking apprehensive. The adult you begins to feel a great concern for her, inviting her to sit with you on the bench and getting her out of the sun. You begin to question her about her feelings and why she is looking so upset.

Take some time here and allow your inner child to tell you why she feels unhappy and apprehensive. You may be surprised by her answers.

When you feel she has given you the answers you are looking for, ask her what she needs to feel better. You are now able to comfort her and rationalize some of her reasons. You tell her she no longer has to worry about these concerns, as you are now in her life and will take care of her. Offer her what she is looking for whether that is a hug, recognition, comfort or security. She is immediately relieved by you and your attempts to comfort her. You both smile at each other and you see her happy face, smiling and looking young and peaceful. Take time now enjoying the youthful joy of your inner child.

In time, she gets up from the bench and leaves you skipping and hopping as a happy child does and you both wave till she is out of your sight. You are left feeling content and happy and get up from the bench and come back into your space by opening your eyes. You now feel comfortable that you can meet with your inner child whenever you feel her vulnerabilities and feel confident that you have the power to help her now. Meet with her often and become her best friend. This will give her less reason to act out and manipulate your adult life.

Affirmations to Gain Back Your Power and Control
I am in control of my body and my life
I believe in myself

Psychotherapy to Assist Your Understanding of Yourself
Work on issues pertaining to low self-esteem and improving your personal boundaries.

Hands-On-Healing Exercise for Candida
Work through the solar plexus chakra, the seat of self-esteem and containing the pancreas. Practice sitting quietly at least once a day, keeping your hands raised about six inches over the solar plexus area in the middle of the abdomen. Maintain for ten to twenty minutes, feeling the sensations change. Before you end, imagine a vivid yellow light moving outward from your solar plexus into the space surrounding your whole body, covering you in a protective yellow mist that will maintain your personal boundaries in a loving and appropriate way, and protect and contain your own energy.

Insulin Resistance

Women who are overweight can go through life feeling shame, guilt and blame for not being able to control their weight, resulting in the loss of their confidence and the destruction of their self-esteem. For them, the recognition of the condition, insulin resistance, brings some relief and justification to their silent battle with their bodies. Insulin resistance, also known as syndrome X or metabolic syndrome, explains why some overweight women find it harder to control their appetites and easier to gain weight than others. Mostly being unaware of this underlying condition, women come for help with depression, eating disorders, digestive problems and for weight issues only to later discover that they may actually have insulin resistance, and leaving with more understanding of their weight and appetite. Not all women with insulin resistance are obese, some are only slightly overweight, but display a pot belly and broad waistline, seemingly disproportionate for their weight, while a few are of normal weight. What most of them have in common is their frustration with putting on weight no matter what they eat or how much they exercise and their complaint of a ravenous appetite that seems impossible to satisfy. They all express their love of carbohydrates and, as they talk about the bread, cakes, cookies, pies, tacos, pizza and sandwiches they eat, I can hear in their voices an overly zealous passion rising, as if powered by an addiction. They talk of their exhilaration at eating food and their fatigue, discomfort, anxiety and depression, often following food. But mostly they express the fear and frustration that they have no control over their food consumption, their weight and their lives.

Physical

In insulin resistance, the pancreatic hormone, insulin, finds it harder to transport glucose from the blood stream into the cells so energy can be made. What this creates is a situation where there are long periods where the blood stream is full of glucose, having no where to go and cells desperate for glucose. Many signals are generated to rectify this situation, all having their part in the development and progression of insulin resistance. As the blood stream sits full of glucose, a misguided signal is perceived that there is too much glucose available, putting metabolism in a fat storing mode and producing women with a sluggish metabolism that is resistant to weight loss. The other problem simultaneously occurring is that the cells are looking for glucose and sending their own message to the brain to delay the satiety message in the hope of getting glucose through more food consumption. This can diminish the ability of women to feel satisfied from their food and increases the risk of overeating. This is often what causes women to crave something sweet, like chocolate, even after eating a full meal or, for some, to have to eat unusually large amounts in order to generate a sense of fullness. The next remedial action to occur, that can push women more toward an insulin resistant state, is that the pancreas is stimulated into producing more insulin in the hope of getting glucose into the cells. Sometimes the amount of insulin needed to get glucose into the cells is many times greater than should be necessary, creating a state of hyper-insulimia. Higher levels of insulin in the blood stream are, again, a signal that glucose is abundant and needs storing, resulting in more fat storage and making it even harder for women to control their weight. As an evolutionary adaptation, these mechanisms are all protective in nature, with insulin increasing the storage of fat for those times when food is unavailable. This may have helped in the days when food was less available and you did not know when your next meal would be, but in this present time of food abundance and with such a great reduction in physical activity to acquire food, this mechanism is only adding to increasing levels of obesity and the rise of insulin resistance. In women's health, the growth of fat cells brings further problems as they have the capacity to make estrogen, upsetting hormonal balance and causing many common hormonal conditions, such as polycystic ovary syndrome, breast cancer, endometrial cancer, candida, endometriosis and fibroids. High levels of insulin can also cause hormone imbalance through the kidneys and liver, generating cardiovascular symptoms, such as hypertension, high cholesterol and increased triglyceride levels, increasing the risk of hardening of the arteries, Alzheimer's disease and liver disease. With a blood stream full with glucose, women can find themselves more open to candida, acne and thrush, as sugar in the blood feeds living organisms; and at risk for developing arthritis, infections and digestive problems, as the sugar creates an unhealthy acidic state. But probably the most serious risk in insulin resistance is that the pancreas will eventually become exhausted by producing so much insulin, resulting in type II diabetes and all its complications.

Emotional

Looking beyond the physical steps that lead to insulin resistance, we can find answers that are more about the women themselves than their body's metabolism. The stories behind the lives of those with insulin resistance usually contain years of emotional stress and a deep sadness, something you can see in the droop of their shoulders, the hesitance in their walk or the layers of clothes they hide behind. Their bodies are showing the signs that stress hormones have been dominating their lives, with the accumulation of large pockets of fat around their abdomen and wrinkles on their brow that hold their permanent frowns. Internally, these women are facing an even bigger battle, as their long-term dependence on stress hormones cause an even greater stress as their bodies have to cope with the opposing forces of insulin (which stores energy) and the stress hormones (which use large amounts of it). Through the high levels of cortisol produced in stress, the uptake of glucose into the cells is slowed to preserve glucose levels for the great demands of stress. To facilitate this preservation mechanism, the long-term actions of the stress hormone, noradrenalin, slowly reduce the cells' ability to take up insulin. Through both of these compensatory activities of the stress hormones, insulin's beneficial functions are reduced while trying to protect women from their stressful lives, resulting in the condition of insulin resistance. Unfortunately, as stress causes the dominance of stress hormones, the ability of insulin to maintain blood sugar is lost, only adding to the emotional instability of these women. Weight and food issues become compounded by an underlying presence of depression, which is often common in women with insulin resistance and cause lower than normal levels of serotonin. In the body's great desire to fight off depression, it will try to make more serotonin to balance this deficit by increasing cravings for carbohydrates that contain the amino acid, tryptophan, the building block from which serotonin is made. This only gives more power to their food cravings and increases their struggle with their bodies, moods and lives.

Spiritual

Underlying this depression and lack of control in their lives, insulin resistant women have a deep sense of emptiness and hopelessness that is rooted in their low self-esteem. Somewhere within their young lives they have picked up the feeling that they did not matter, creating a void within themselves that becomes hard to fill. They become driven by the great need to fill this emptiness by justifying their existence and making themselves feel deserving, using food as one of their tools. Instead of responding to food in a normal way, all their energy and motivation is geared into filling their void, causing them to override all their innate feeding reflexes to get their ultimate need met. This causes detachment, not only from the signals of their bodies, but also from their higher selves. With the loss of their own self-awareness, they also lose the ability to take in nourishment properly and the message that the cells receive is that they are not worthy to be feed, nourished or loved, and they too begin to resist nourishment by impeding insulin's actions. Unconsciously, these women over-compensate for their emptiness by desperately trying to fill themselves up with fast acting carbo-hydrates in an attempt to satisfy their needs. Their lives become as distorted as their bodies, as they find it hard to find value in their existence and their cells respond accordingly, reducing the avail-ability of energy to them. There is often a sense of desperation in these women, with the unmet needs of their early lives moving them in one direction, and the needs of their body moving them in another. With their physical and spiritual needs both moving in different directions, the void only becomes bigger, creating more detachment, despair and hunger. The more they feed themselves, the sicker they get, and the more unresponsive their insulin becomes. The bigger their bodies grow in size, the stronger their message becomes, saying 'Here I am. See me, feed me, love me'.

Nutritional Healing in Insulin Resistance

The main issue in the diet for insulin resistance is to remove sugar from the diet. Because insulin resistance can cause both hypoglycemia and hyperglycemia, women with insulin resistance remain a victim to their oscillating blood sugar levels if there diet is not controlled. Sugar feeds the symptoms of insulin resistance and makes them more severe and dramatic, generating much more stress in their lives. A blood stream already full of glucose only needs a chocolate bar to signal a stress response and a state of hyperglycemia, sending out adrenalin and moving the body and mind into a stress mode, causing women to feel hyped-up with anxiety, agitation, anger, rage and depression for no apparent reason. The same kind of stress is also felt in hypoglycemia, when excessive insulin causes too rapid a reduction in blood sugar, again signaling the stress response and the same kind of feelings. Women often get used to these ups and downs when they occur regularly and can lose track of how stressful it is to them, learning to live with an uncomfortable level of stress always in their lives. It is usually not until they remove sugar from the diet for at least two weeks and then introduce some, that they can fully appreciate the full extent of their stress, feeling their body, mind and emotions change almost instantly. The good news is that insulin resistance is very manageable through diet and can be reduced just by avoiding sugar and lowing carbohydrate intake.

Diet Management of Insulin Resistance

Reducing Carbohydrates in the Diet

- Avoid all sugars and sugar products, including white sugar, maple syrup, honey, molasses, dried fruits, cookies, candy, cakes, bakery products, processed cereals, fast foods, junk foods, colas, soft drinks and desserts
- Eliminate refined carbohydrates found in bread, cake, cookies, bread crumbs, pasta and processed cereals
- Grains are best avoided, but if eaten should be as whole as possible, such as pinhead oats instead of rolled oats, brown rice instead of white, whole grains instead of processed cereals
- Make carbohydrates a smaller percentage of each meal
- If carbohydrates are eaten, ensure there is fat or protein eaten alongside to slow blood sugar release
- In choosing fruits and vegetables use the glycemic index for the best choices for a slower release into the blood stream. For example, cherries with a glycemic index of 22 and grapefruits at 25 are better choices than bananas at 54 and grapes at 46
- Never skip a meal
- Always eat breakfast and try to make it have the least carbo-hydrates of all meals so that blood sugar has a better regulation through the day
- Eat fruit instead of fruit juice as fiber is beneficial to blood sugar

- Eat foods high in omega 3, essential fatty acids such as avocado, salmon, tuna, herring, mackerel, sardines, flax seeds, pumpkin seeds and eggs to improve metabolism

Foods that Help in the Management of Insulin Resistance
- Meats
- Fish
- Poultry
- Eggs
- Live unsweetened yogurt
- Nut and seeds
- Beans and legumes
- Leafy green vegetables

Supplements Helpful in Insulin Resistance
- Magnesium 400mg a day to reduce insulin resistance and help depression
- B-complex 50 to improve metabolism and nerve and brain functions
- Vitamin C 500mg with bioflavonoid twice a day for endocrine health
- Chromium 50mcg a day to support blood sugar levels
- Zinc 20mg a day to support the endocrine system and balance blood sugar

Physical Exercise for Insulin Resistance
I am going to have to add exercise here as it is invaluable to the treatment of insulin resistance. Exercise increases the amount of oxygen getting in to cells, reducing insulin resistance and increasing metabolism. With exercise there is a reduction in the dominance of stress hormones, an increase in serotonin and endorphins, improving mood and self-confidence. There is no better addition to the management strategy of insulin resistance than including walking, swimming, cycling, running, tai chi, yoga

or dancing to your daily routine.

Herbal Healing of Insulin Resistance

Aims of Herbal Treatment for Insulin Resistance
Balance Blood Sugar
Sacred basil, cinnamon, goats rue, gurmar, bilberry, globe artichoke, dandelion root, fringe tree, nettle leaf, alfalfa

Support the Pancreas and Liver to Improve Metabolism and Digestion
Fringe tree, dandelion root, globe artichoke, milk thistle, iris, barberry, Oregon grape root, burdock

Support Adrenal Glands and Reduce Stress and Cortisol Levels
Siberian ginseng, borage, schisandra, gotu kola, astragalus, licorice, ashwaghanda.

Reduce Anxiety, Tension and Depression
Skullcap, betony, vervain, valerian, oats, St.John's wort, pulsatilla, damiana, passionflower, rose, chamomile, rosemary, lavender.

Examples of Herbal Remedies for Insulin Resistance
Insulin Resistance with Obesity and Food Cravings

Sacred basil	15ml	Balances blood sugar
Goats rue	20ml	Balances blood sugar
Gurmar	5ml	Reduces taste for sugar
Fringe tree	20ml	Support pancreatic function
Licorice	15ml	Adrenal gland tonic, anti-stress
St. John's wort	<u>25ml</u>	Improves well-being
	100ml	

Dose: 5ml (one teaspoon) three times a day

Insulin Resistance with Mood Problems (depression, anxiety, irritability)

Dandelion root	15ml	Balances blood sugar
Bilberry	**20ml**	**Balances blood sugar**
Gurmar	**5ml**	**Reduces taste for sugar**
Borage	20ml	Adrenal tonic
Skullcap	20ml	Emotional balancer
Rose	<u>20ml</u>	Improves well-being
	100ml	

Dose: 5ml (one teaspoon) three times a day

Insulin Resistance with Estrogen Dominance Reproductive Conditions (endometriosis, fibroids, premenstrual syndrome, breast cancer)

Nettle leaf	15ml	Balances blood sugar
Gurmar	5ml	Reduces taste for sugar
Fringe tree	20ml	Balances blood sugar
Gotu kola	25ml	Support adrenal glands
Vervain	20ml	Relaxing nerve tonic
Pulsatilla	<u>15ml</u>	Anti-stress and reduces pain
	100ml	

Dose: 5ml (one teaspoon) three times a day

Insulin Resistance with Candida

Cinnamon	20ml	Balances blood sugar
Gurmar	5ml	Reduces taste for sugar
Oregon grape root	15ml	Cleanse digestive system
Ashwaghanda	25ml	Anti-stress, relaxing
Betony	20ml	Relaxing nerve tonic
Chamomile	<u>15ml</u>	Calming to digestion
	100ml	

Dose: 5ml (one teaspoon) three times a day

Healing Tools for Insulin Resistance

Aims of healing

- Develop self-love

- Improve self-esteem
- Learn to nurture and care for oneself

Meditation for Insulin Resistance
This meditation will help women become more aware of themselves and help to fill the emptiness they feel inside.

Wake up earlier so you can give yourself an extra twenty to thirty minutes to sit in meditation. Find a space that is quiet, so you will be undisturbed. Close your eyes and direct your attention inwards, becoming aware of the way you are breathing. With your mouth closed, feel the air moving into your nose with your in-breath, feel your diaphragm expanding and then contracting with the out-breath and feel it pass out through your nose again. Follow your breathing for a few minutes, becoming familiar with it, feeling yourself drift into its rhythm.

Begin to hum after the out-breath and with each out-breath feel the sound vibrating through your mouth, throat and voice box. Repeat until you get a rhythm.

As you continue, allow the sound to vibrate into your body, filling its space before ending. After a while you may find you cannot separate yourself from the sound. When this occurs wander into the unbound space that surrounds you, letting your mind and body drift and stop the humming sound. With your mind and body still, just enjoy the feeling of being in this space. If you lose sight of it, go back to your humming until you find it again.

When you feel you have achieved a sense of peace and relaxation, after about twenty to thirty minutes, open your eyes and sit for a few minutes feeling your tranquility. Feel how comfortable you are in your own body. The more this meditation is done, the closer you will become to your own energy and the more you will have reduced your emptiness.

Visualization for Insulin Resistance

Create an image of yourself of how you would like to look. Maybe it's the way you looked when you were happier, or the way you have felt when you had more confidence. Visualize the clothes you would wear, the style of your hair and the way you would stand tall. Keep this image always in your mind and think about it throughout your day. See it when you first wake up in the morning and make it your last thought before sleep. In time, your body will move you towards this image.

Inner Child Visualization for Insulin Resistance

There is an inner child in many women with insulin resistance, who needs to know they are valuable, important and worth caring for. Although their needs may not have been met in their developing years, there are still ways they can learn to accept, nurture and love themselves, instead of waiting for someone else to do so. The following exercise will help develop a relationship with the inner child.

Find a quiet and peaceful space and play relaxing background music. Sit comfortably with your feet touching the floor and enjoy the tranquility, as the music fills the room. Take three deep breaths, big enough to release the tension, anxiety and stress in your body. Sit for a moment and feel the restfulness of your body and mind as it unwinds.

Begin to picture yourself getting ready for a gentle walk on a sunny spring day. See yourself closing the door behind you, and as you turn around and step out, you are transported into a beautiful green field of wild flowers humming with the energy of spring. The sun is shining warmly and there is the gentlest of breezes making you feel comfortable. The field is dotted with white daisies and yellow dandelions, and the intoxicating scent of spring is in the air, making you feel its lifting energy all around you. You can hear the soft whispers of different birds busy in their nesting activity. As you walk along, entranced by the tranquility, you become aware of a positive energy within you. You see yourself smiling, as you take in the beauty that surrounds you. Continue walking and enjoy the serenity, feel your body getting more relaxed and your mood soaring.

In the distance you notice a huge, old, oak tree its branches moving out in all directions. As you approach the tree, you see there is an opening, large enough to sit in. It seems friendly and your adventurous spirit calls for you to make your way in and sit on its dry mossy seat. An overwhelming feeling of safety takes over you as you relax comfortably into the hollow of the tree. Enjoy this feeling of comfort for a few minutes, as your body relaxes into its welcoming embrace and the smell of the earth fills you with comfort.

You begin to hear the steps of someone walking towards the tree. As you peer out you see a little girl. You recognize her as yourself at a very young age. Take some time to visualize yourself at an age of vulnerability and slowly see yourself become the little girl that stands in front of you.

She seems insecure and hesitant, but you coax her in to sit with you. The two of you sit there facing each other. You begin asking her what is wrong and why she looks so upset. See yourself speaking gently to her and wait to hear her response. Take time here and allow her to speak to you.

When she answers you, you are able to give her what she needs. You are the only person in her life that can offer her the support and *soul-utions* to her problems. If she needs a hug, give her a hug. If she needs to be held, hold her. If she needs to cry, allow her the space. Make her aware of your commitment to help her. She now has no more need to feel alone or empty, as you will be watching over her. Ask her if she would like to come home with you so you can care for her. Tell her you will make sure she is fed, clean and loved. You will make sure she has everything she needs.

Take her hand as you leave the tree. Walk with her, hand and hand and lead her back the way you came. Both of you are feeling happy as you stroll in the sun. There is a lightness in both of you and she begins to skip and sing joyfully as only an innocent child can. As you approach your front door and put the key in, you welcome her into your home.

Take your time enjoying the space the two of you share. See her happy and content in this new home. When you are ready, become aware of the background music and bring your focus back into the room and open your eyes.

Continue to spend time with your inner child and get close to her, allowing her to feel comfortable and safe with you. Bring her walking with you, have her in the car with you and learn to nurture her as she deserves. See her always smiling and happy and you will find yourself a much happier person with less food issues.

Affirmations for insulin resistance
    I believe in myself
    I deserve to care for myself
    I am a valuable part of life

Psychotherapy for Insulin Resistance
    Work on issues surrounding self-esteem

Hands-On-Healing Exercise for Insulin Resistance
Whenever you are sitting quietly and relaxed, take time to be aware of your abdomen area, which contains the solar plexus chakra and is the space needing filling and nurturing. Raise your hands about six inches above your abdominal area and keep them there for ten to fifteen minutes at a time. Every so often, draw a deep breath and bring it down into the solar plexus. As breath is drawn down, feel the color yellow grow stronger and wider within the abdominal cavity, filling it with a warm nurturing, until you feel as if you are containing the sun within your solar plexus and enjoying the feelings of confidence and power it brings.

Premenstrual Syndrome

There is probably no more compelling female hormonal condition than premenstrual syndrome. For anyone that has not experienced its intense turbulence during their cycle, it is hard to appreciate just how destructive it can be in women's lives. In a period of one week, women that suffer with premenstrual syndrome can go through dramatic changes that alter their physical body, emotional stability and the way they perceive the world around them. Their weight can alter, their facial expressions are modified, the type of clothes they wear change, the foods they eat are different, their relationships become more difficult, their behavior seems odd, and their lives just do not feel right anymore. Then, just when they reach their lowest ebb, a relieving change occurs and most of the anguish is forgotten until the next turn of the cycle. It's a terrifying experience that is repeated over again during many women's cycles, bringing self-loathing, confusion, destruction and exhaustion in its wake. What is so intriguing in premenstrual syndrome is that women adamantly refuse to accept the negativity that comes up during this phase as part of themselves, preferring to believe they have a 'hormonal problem', eliminating much of their personal responsibility; no one wants to believe there is so much darkness within themselves. The sadness of premenstrual syndrome is that it is so destructive, that without women getting the right kind of help, they continually hurt the people around them and are always left with a sense of self-loathing, over and over again.

Physical

There are many physiological reasons why women feel different during the luteal phase and most of them have to do with its dominate hormone, progesterone. Starting as early as day fifteen and ending as late as day twenty-six of the menstrual cycle, women begin to feel changes within themselves as progesterone rises and estrogen is lowered, bringing physical and mental changes to women at varying individual levels. When estrogen is lowered, women lose the physical and mental energy it brings, along with the stimulation of the neurotransmitters, dopamine, noradrenalin and serotonin, which follows its decline. Rising progesterone, on the other hand, brings a slowness to mental and physical processes as it promotes the rise of inhibiting neurotransmitters, such as gamma amino butyric acid (GABA). The conclusion of both these developments cause women, during the luteal phase, to be more vulnerable to low energy, poor stamina, slowness in thought, lowered concentration, clumsiness, forgetfulness, be accident prone and open to depression. This same mechanism has an affect on immune function, where estrogen increases immunity and progesterone reduces it, causing the luteal phase to be a time of lower immune function for women, and a reason many women experiences relapses of illnesses such as cystitis, thrush, eczema, asthma and colds during this phase. Progesterone dominance in this phase also naturally causes an increase in carbohydrate metabolism, an evolutionary mechanism that maintained women's weight if conception occurred. However, without conception, this rise in blood sugar can cause women great dips in blood sugar, causing hypoglycemia and leaving them with more hunger, weight gain, fatigue, headaches, migraines, breast pains and anxiety. Many of these symptoms can be exaggerated in premenstrual syndrome by the interference of stress hormones or birth control pills, both of which also interfere with blood sugar, making all symptoms more dramatic.

Emotional

Emotional stress is often the power behind premenstrual syndrome and, instead of it being thought of as a hormonal condition, it really should be looked at as a condition of stress. When stressful life experiences are continuous in young girls' and women's lives, they learn to repress their anger, shame and pain by relying on their adrenal glands to produce stress hormones to counteract these emotions and to help them cope with their lives. This mechanism can be especially damaging to young girls around the time of menarche, when their endocrine system is developing a communication between all the glands to create a healthy reproductive system. The habitual production of stress hormones can undermine the hormonal integrity of the endocrine system and later cause conditions such as premenstrual syndrome. The production of stress hormones, particularly cortisol, requires large amounts of a starting material, which is the same that is used for progesterone production. With cortisol being produced in excessive amounts to meet the demands of stressful lives, the amount of progesterone that is able to be produced is lessened. With lower levels of progesterone, estrogen is inappropriately forced into dominating a phase that progesterone should, creating an exaggerated sense of stimulation in a phase that is very inward looking. Emotions get out of hand in premenstrual syndrome when women, highly charged with estrogen, aggressively confront their repressed emotions, which become more accessible to them during this inward-looking phase. What adds drama to this already volatile phase is an unsteady blood sugar, looking for large amounts of carbohydrates to comfort rising emotions, which only result in greater agitation, nervousness, restlessness, confusion, mania, aggression and rage. But what actually causes women with premenstrual syndrome to be unable to tolerate their lives during the luteal phase is their underlying emotional pain which they can no longer hide.

Spiritual

On a spiritual level, premenstrual syndrome is interesting because it occurs during the phase when women's most profound feminine hormone, progesterone, becomes dominate. There is no other hormone that brings women closer to their female nature than progesterone, producing changes in the body enabling women to bear children and supporting the instincts that enable motherhood. Many women tell of their particularly bad bout of premenstrual syndrome following a period of time when they have lost track of their own space and energy, giving themselves up to others around them, which happens so easily to women in their caring roles as mothers, wives, sisters and daughters. So when their nurturing hormone, progesterone begins rising, reminding them of their female responsibilities during the luteal phase, there will be resentment and resistance to these energies. All the times they should have said 'no' instead of 'yes' during the last month have been building up, and now, without the defenses of the other phases, one little 'no' now has the power to become a wild outburst containing all the anger, resentment and vengeance they have been holding back. Very often, this is fed by a deep wound to their female image, growing up in homes where they are unable to feel good about their female role models, some confused by their actions, others finding it hard to trust them, some rejected by them, and still others made to feel inadequate by them. These wounds create an unconscious rejection of their female hormone, progesterone, and their feminine roles and qualities which rise forward in the luteal phase. With the rise of progesterone at this time also come alterations in neurotransmitters, which initiate a strong inward focus, causing them to feel more than is usually accessible during the other phases, and allowing the resentment and anger of their wounds to resurface with an intensity. The rejection of progesterone not only hurts those around them, but limits their own female potential by blocking the energy that brings them their creative and intuitive nature.

Nutritional Healing in Premenstrual Syndrome

The most helpful dietary advice in premenstrual syndrome is to control the amount of simple sugars in the diet to avoid hypoglycemia which can trigger many premenstrual symptoms. Hypoglycemia can bring on the gluttonous appetite of premenstrual syndrome which ruins all attempts of dieting and weight control. It can make women irritable if they do not get their food fast enough and then tired after eating so much. It can cause lose of concentration before food and headaches after food. There may be restlessness before a meal and depression or rage after one. Due to the natural changes that progesterone makes to blood sugar, simple sugars, in some women, can become their nemesis and cause the aggressive and dramatic changes in personality that make women feel so desperate in premenstrual syndrome.

Diet Management for Premenstrual Syndrome
Avoid Hypoglycemia
- Eat proteins and fats at breakfast to sustain blood sugar throughout day
- Eat less carbohydrates and increase proteins, especially poultry, fish, eggs, nuts and seeds
- Avoid all sugar and sugar products, including white sugar, maple syrup, honey, molasses, cookies, candy, cakes, processed cereals, fast foods, processed foods, colas, juices, soft drinks and desserts
- Eat from foods low in the GI index
- Increase high fiber foods to help improve blood sugar
- Avoid stimulants in coffee, tea, alcohol, chocolate, which cause mood swings
- Do not skip any meals
- Have high protein snacks always available, like nuts and

seeds, for a quick snack and to prevent hunger
- Organize your own food for each day and cook it yourself

Supplements for Premenstrual Syndrome
- Magnesium 400mg a day to help keep emotional stability
- Chromium to balance blood sugar
- B-complex Vitamins to improve blood sugar and metabolism
- Vitamin C and bioflavonoids to reduce stress

Herbal Healing for Premenstrual Syndrome

The great mistake most people make when trying to treat their premenstrual syndrome with herbs is thinking of it as a hormonal condition and using hormonally active herbs that only cause more disorder. Most of what women experience premenstrually is not directly coming from the reproductive organs, but more of a consequence of imbalances on many different levels. It is vitally important to help women relax and to reduce the stress in their lives so they can cope better with their premenstrual changes. This, along with control over their blood sugar, can be an enormous help in reducing symptoms. Then we can begin to look at the symptoms which are most uncomfortable and treat them, such as water retention, headaches, irritable bowel and depression. There is great relief with the use of herbs in premenstrual syndrome when they are used appropriately and with the individual woman in mind and not the condition.

Aims of Herbal Treatment for Premenstrual Syndrome
Relax the Body and Mind
Skullcap, vervain, betony, St. John's wort, oats, rose, valerian, anemone, chamomile, linden blossoms, lavender

Improve Adrenal Gland Function and Increase Ability to Cope with Stress

Siberian ginseng, gotu kola, ashwaghanda, astragalus, schisandra, borage

Balance Blood Sugar and Reduce Hypoglycemia
Cinnamon, goats rue, gurmar, bilberry, globe artichoke, dandelion root, fringe tree

Balance Endocrine Function through the Pituitary Gland
Chaste tree

Treat any Uncomfortable Symptoms, Such as Bloating, Water Retention or Depression
For appropriate herbs see below

Examples of Herbal Remedies for Premenstrual Syndrome
Premenstrual Syndrome with Anxiety, Irritability and Mood Swing

Skullcap	30ml	Emotional balancer, nerve tonic
Ashwaghanda	25ml	Anti-stress, relaxing to nerves
Goats rue	20ml	Balances blood sugar
Gurmar	5ml	Reduces taste for sugar
Valerian	20m	Natural tranquillizer
	100ml	

Dose 5ml (one teaspoon) three times a day, throughout cycle

Premenstrual Syndrome with Food Cravings and Weight Gain

Betony	30ml	Relaxing nerve tonic
Siberian Ginseng	15ml	Anti-stress
Cinnamon	20ml	Balances blood sugar
Gurmar	5ml	Reduces taste for sugar
Fringe Tree	15ml	Balances blood sugar
Chamomile	15ml	Calming to the nerves
	100ml	

Dose 5ml (one teaspoon) three times a day, throughout cycle

Premenstrual Syndrome with Depression

Oats	20ml	Anti-depressant, nerve balancer
Gotu kola	20ml	Anti-stress
Dandelion root	20ml	Balances blood sugar, tonic
St. John's wort	20ml	Anti-depressant
Rose	20ml	Improve self-esteem
	100ml	

Dose 5ml (one teaspoon) three times a day, throughout cycle

Premenstrual Syndrome with Water Retention, Sore Breasts and Irregular Periods

Vervain	20ml	Relaxing nerve tonic
Astragalus	20ml	Kidney tonic, anti-stress
Globe artichoke	20ml	Improves blood sugar
Dandelion leaf	15ml	Reduces water retention
Linden blossoms	20ml	Soothing to nerves
Chaste tree	5ml	Endocrine balancer
	100ml	

Dose 5ml (one teaspoon) three times a day, throughout cycle

Healing Tools for Premenstrual Syndrome

Aims of Healing
- Giving oneself time and space
- Learning to relax the body and mind
- Accepting all aspects of oneself

Meditation for Premenstrual Syndrome

Meditation offers women with premenstrual syndrome the time and space they need to revive and reconnect with themselves. With practice, it can reduce resentment, stop depletion, foster relaxation and retain anonymity, all helping to improve their female image of themselves.

Sitting in a quiet room, where you will not be disturbed, sit with your feet touching the floor and your back firmly supported. Close your eyes and become aware of your breath, focusing on each in-breath and out-breath. You are now going to start to count from ten to one, very slowly and deliberating, taking time with each individual number, seeing it appear in your mind in bold type, as if on a blackboard. Keep saying to yourself that with each number you will become more and more relaxed, so that by the time you reach one, your body is calm and your mind restful. As each number appears in your mind, see the white of the number and be aware of the black space surrounding it. Close everything else out of your mind and just focus on the number as it becomes a vivid image in your mind. Feel a sense of relaxation come over you with each number. If your mind wanders, bring it back to the numbers and start counting again from ten downwards. It may take a few rounds of numbers to feel the restfulness that helps you drift into meditation. Each time number one is reached, you should feel like allowing your mind to drift into a meditative state. Try to sit in this empty space for 20 to 30 minutes. As you do more of this exercise, it will become easier for you to go into meditation.

When you are finished, open your eyes and sit with your eyes open for a while, bringing your body and mind gently back.

Visualization to Help Increase Relaxation in Premenstrual Syndrome
Women who get premenstrual syndrome are usually stressed and overwhelmed by their lives. Their body and mind have become used to running on stress hormones, leaving them easily exhausted and often intolerant. They usually work very hard, do things fast, and are usually just waiting for something to go wrong; always living their lives in anticipation of danger, a legacy of their stress hormones. To reduce this dependence on their sympathetic nervous system, it is immensely helpful to have them take twenty to thirty minutes a day in quiet visualization that can bring their body and mind back to balance and help them

rely more on the parasympathetic nervous system.

Appoint a time in your day when you can give yourself this space. In a peaceful room, close your eyes and take a few deep breaths, breathing out tension and breathing in peace. Become aware of your breath and follow it for a few minutes, allowing the mind and body to relax. Start to imagine a place in a landscape where you have been happy, relaxed, safe and joyful on your own. If you cannot think of such a place, make one up. It can be in a garden, on a beach, by a waterfall, on top of a mountain, or hidden deep within a mossy forest. But what's important is to actually feel the sunshine on you, the wind brush your cheek or hear the sound of the leaves rustling under your feet. Make sure you can smell the scent of flowers or the salty sea air, hear the birds chirping or the wind through the trees; feel your body as it lies over warm sand or a carpet of newly mowed lawn. Sense how your body begins to become more relaxed as your images get stronger, your muscles become less tense and your mind becomes restful. You feel peaceful in this place and you begin to feel a sense of enthusiastic joy come over you. See yourself looking around and smiling, humming or laughing. Allow yourself as much time as you like in this place. As you practice this restful visualization, you will get better at it, go deeper each time, and more easily give up to its intoxicating gripe. Not only will you be giving yourself a physical rest, but you will be reducing the power of emotions and becoming more familiar with yourself.

Inner Child Work for Premenstrual Syndrome
Go through old photographs of yourself as a child. There is usually one you respond to strongly; it could be one you took at school, or one with a look on it that makes you remember a part of yourself long gone, or one that makes you anxious. Keep this image in your mind and one day, when alone, relaxed and in a place that feels safe, whether it is in a bath, sitting by a lake, sitting under a tree or in the safety of your bedroom, bring it up clearly

in your mind. Start by taking some deeps breaths, breathing out any negative thoughts and breathing in clean, fresh space for a new possibilities. Visualize your inner child as she was in the photo. See her image become clear and vivid in your mind. You may begin to feel good emotions or bad ones, but allow them to come forward. Begin a dialogue with your inner child and try to find out some of the reasons she may be unhappy or worried.

Now from the perspective of your older self today, try to explain to her how you see these situations and why they may have occurred. As you explain this to her, see her face begin to smile and change with reassurance. The face in the photo now begins to take a different feeling, remaining in your mind as one of a joyful enthusiastic child, with few cares and worries. Let her image fade with this thought in your mind. Whenever you visualize the photo again, always see her smiling and happy. Do this exercise as often as possible, bringing up her photo in your mind and ensuring it brings up a child-like joy.

Affirmations for Premenstrual Syndrome

I believe and trust in myself

I deserve kindness, caring and feeling safe

I value my female nature

Psychotherapy in Premenstrual Syndrome

Women who suffer with premenstrual syndrome should explore with a psychotherapist aspects of their shadow side, the dark part of themselves that they are uncomfortable with and which they often repress. It is this part of themselves that becomes active during the luteal phase and which they have repressed so deeply that, when it comes forward, they are surprised by its presence and its power. These are the parts of themselves they need to recognize and become more familiar with so they become a more positive force in their lives than a negative one.

Hands-On-Healing Exercise for Premenstrual Syndrome
When wounds occur during the formative years of 5 to 8 years old, when young girls are building images of themselves as women, their wounds can have a potency affecting not only their femininity, but also their sexuality and their creativity. Premenstrual syndrome gets its power from the repression of these powerful forces. Freeing up the energy in the sacral chakra allows for women to experience their true nature through the spontaneity of their child-like nature from which is built a healthy image of their femininity, a playful sexuality, and an impulsive creativity.

Become familiar with your sacral chakra by placing your hands over the area which is between the bellybutton and the pelvic bone. Hold your hands about six inches above this area and stay in that position for ten to fifteen minutes at a time trying to pick up its energy. See if it feels warm, cold, blocked, stagnate or turbulent. Be aware of the changes you feel in yourself.

Before you end, take some deep breaths and breathe down into this space bringing fresh, positive energy. As you breathe, the color in the sacral area becomes more orange with each breath. Feel the color enclosing the sacral space and feel the energy change to one of comfort and strength. Leave with the thought that you have brought some peace and balance to the energy of your sacral chakra. Before taking your hands away, contain this good energy by imaging the orange petals of a marigold flower covering over this orange energy and containing it with only a hint of orange light peeking through the petals, preserving the energy of your femininity, sexuality and creativity.

The Keeping of a Moon Diary
One of the most valuable tools for women with premenstrual syndrome is the keeping of a moon diary to help chart the changing rhythms of their cycle and to be able to visualize their changing ways more easily. Its very much like the keeping of a

diary only this time it's in a circular pattern. Each month take a large piece of paper and draw a circle trying to fill the whole of the paper. Divide the circle up into twenty-eight to thirty sections, or as many as the length of your normal cycle. Number each section by day, starting the first day you bleed as day one and continuing through to the end of the cycle. Start the second moon diary on the day you start to bleed again. On each circle note the phase of the moon on the day you bleed and also at your ovulation by either drawing a full or dark moon, or writing it in. In the section of each day, write in the most significant feelings in the day, whether it has to do with moods, feelings, energy level, food habits, sleep patterns, dreams, relationships, headaches, health, stress levels, mucus secretions, etc. Anything that can best describe the significance of that day for you.

In the first month you will not have anything to compare this to, so it will not mean much to you. The second month you will have two months, which may begin to show you some interesting coincidences. But by the third month you will begin to see a pattern in your changing body, emotions and spirit: this is your changing nature. What occurs through keeping a moon diary is that you begin to see patterns in your behavior, moods and physical health that you normally do not recognize. By acknowledging them you can begin to appreciate your changing ways and become more accepting of yourself. You know when you go down, you will come up again, and you know when you cannot concentrate on your work, it will come back again. Becoming aware of your changing ways makes life less difficult and keeps you from being hard on yourself. You can also begin to see your cycle having more benefits than disadvantages. Instead of trying to have a party during your bleeding time, when you feel you would rather be alone, choose to make it the week after your period, when you are feeling more social. When you have to make big decisions in your life, wait until your menstrual phase for inspiration and intuition to help in your decision making. When you have to confront someone and want to let them down gently, do it when ovulating, when the chances of hurting someone is lessened. Instead of starting a diet during your luteal phase, wait until your follicular phase, when your blood sugar is more balanced.

It's also interesting to see how your own phases compare to the phases of the moon, bringing a greater connection and a deeper understanding of the cycles of nature. Through the moon diary comes acceptance, understanding, forgiveness and self-love. You will no longer fall down into the depths of self-hatred after a premenstrual rage, or call yourself derogatory names for forgetting an appointment. It will show you your best days and your worst days, your masculine energies and your feminine energies and bring self-discovery and acceptance, reducing the symptoms of premenstrual syndrome.

(This idea was adapted from a lovely book by Mirandra Grey, The Red Moon: Understanding and Using the Gifts of the Menstrual Cycle, which is highly recommended for those looking for greater understanding into their cycle.)

Polycystic Ovary Syndrome

Since the advent of the ultrasound, polycystic ovary syndrome is more easily diagnosed and more women are getting answers to their unusual hormonal symptoms. This brings some relief as it is a condition that comes with some of the most difficult symptoms women have to cope with and practitioners have to treat. In many polycystic women there is great frustration as they gain weight, no matter how much they eat; while the advice given on food choices is often negated by the strong carbohydrate cravings that drive the condition. Excessive hair on their upper lips, arms and breasts could cause much embarrassment for women and be very difficult to totally reverse with treatment. The acne of teenagers, appearing just at a time in their lives when they are putting themselves forward into the world, can be hard to treat long-term when they are so desperate for fast results. The disappointment of failed conceptions becomes an emotional issue that sometimes takes president over the hormonal issues, making it challenging for both the patient and the practitioner. The rampant candida that sometimes accompanies polycystic ovary can make many women lose heart in themselves and lose faith in treatment. Polycystic ovary syndrome is a condition very much powered by emotions and in treating it, you also have to treat the women's defensiveness, resentments and disappointments, which are the driving force behind the condition.

Physical

Polycystic ovary syndrome is truly an endocrine condition with disturbances affecting, not only the ovaries (as it name suggests), but also with disruption at the hypothalamus, pituitary, thyroid, pancreas and adrenal glands, all making for a condition with many complications. It is essentially a hormonal imbalance, where too much male androgens are produced in women. Normally, the androgens, androstenedione and testosterone are made in the ovaries, adrenal glands and fat cells and are a normal part of the female hormone profile, but in polycystic ovaries their numbers become excessive and cause imbalance of other hormones, especially estrogen and progesterone. The majority of women with polycystic ovary syndrome have problems with weight, causing its common complication, insulin resistance, to be blamed on the condition. Fat cells produce androgens normally, but when there are more of them, or they grow in size, androgen levels are increased. The androgens that are made by fat cells are able to be converted into testosterone and estrone, the estrogen that competes with ovarian estridiol. Without sufficient estridiol, polycystic women produce ovarian follicles that are unable to mature into proper eggs, forming cysts and preventing ovulation and reducing fertility. Deprived of a functional follicle, many polycystic women are unable to produce the estridiol and progesterone that is needed to produce a healthy cycle, leaving these women more at risk to missed periods, irregular cycles, ovarian pain, difficulty conceiving and repeated miscarriages. On another level, excess estrone and testosterone must also compete for the limited number of the carrier molecule, sex hormone binding globulin (SHBG), which enables them to produce their desired effects in the appropriate tissue. Without the aid of this carrier molecule, testosterone circulates alone in the blood stream, without its buffering affects and instead of getting the benefits of testosterone such as stamina, muscle strength, confidence and a healthy sexuality, it produces undesirable masculine features in women, such as excessive hair growth on the upper lip, male patterned baldness at the top of head and pot bellies. It can be the cause of young women getting acne as teenage boys do, when testosterone levels rise causing the glands of the skin to enlarge and excrete excessive oil. Because this condition can also cause estrogen to move through the blood steam without a carrier molecule and cause less receptor availability at its target tissues, it can leave women open to estrogen dominant conditions such as endometriosis, fibroids and reproductive cancers. The level of hormone dysfunction in polycystic ovary syndrome can leave women open to much emotional distress.

Emotional

In a condition with so many physical and emotional issues attached to it, it becomes necessary to seek a common origin so that treatment becomes more healing than interfering. When dealing with hormones, treating symptoms instead of the condition can bring more hormonal complications and is especially relevant with this condition. Looking more closely behind all the complexity of hormones in polycystic ovary syndrome, there is one common feature which stands out and which needs more careful consideration: insulin resistance. Through insulin resistance and its accompanying hyperinsulimia, excessive androgens are produced, making this process an important issue in the development of polycystic ovary syndrome. As we have seen previously, the hormones responsible for the development of insulin resistance are the stress hormones, noradrenalin and cortisol; the same ones young girls and women learn to use to cope with lives that are unsatisfactory, unsafe or unhappy. Through their overuse, physiological changes are initiated that can cause the development of insulin resistance. The continual presence of noradrenalin causes changes at the cell membranes that slow the easy access of insulin, and the chronically high levels of cortisol cause more insulin to be produced. Through long-term stress the body tries to conserve its resources by maintaining a tighter control over blood sugar to cope with a heighten state of stimulation, and insulin resistance is its protective result. To add to the discomfort involved in polycystic ovary syndrome, when women eat foods high in sugar, they can cause a more dramatic state of hyperinsulinemia, resulting in more physical stress with the release of adrenalin only adding to the emotional stress these women feel. With these three stress hormones coursing through their bodies, it is no wonder women with polycystic ovary syndrome appear weary, defensive, aggressive and anxious. Nor is it surprising that many of these girls grow up to become bulimics, with all the charge and intensity of their stress hormones needing release. These are women that need care and to be treated sensitively, even through they seem to be saying, 'leave me alone'.

Spiritual

Polycystic women are women who have had enough. Their hormones confuse them, their bodies are doing the wrong things, they may look different, they feel different and in a very deep way, they *are* different. It is not surprising that they seem hardened in someway, just like their ovaries covered in cysts. Underlying their defensiveness is an unconscious need to protect themselves, caused by a wound to their femininity and one which leads to their rejection of their female nature. The wound could have been caused by sexual abuse, abandonment or rejection by someone they trusted and loved, causing them disappointment, disillusionment, and self-destructiveness. In their outrage, an unconscious decision is made to reject nourishment and all that is female, and there begins a slowing down of their blood sugar, reduction in ovulation and signs of masculine features. With a reduction in female hormones and an increase in male hormones, the energy of polycystic women changes. Instead of blending and balancing each other, to create a physically, emotionally and spiritually healthy women, each of these energies lose their individual positive attributes and become destructive. They lose the joy, optimism and openness that come with ovulation and is replaced by an edgy indifference that can seem hostile, as they try to fend off the aggressive energies of their male hormones. There seems to be a constant conflict always going on inside these women, and even they do not feel comfortable in their own skin, making it easier for organisms, like candida, to take over and become aggressive. Without the unconscious motivation to be well, every-thing is harder for them. Their moods are infected by an erratic blood sugar, their blood sugar is controlled by an irregular cycle, their cycle is managed by imbalanced hormones and in charge of it all is a broken spirit. Without healing the wound at the core of women with polycystic ovary syndrome, there is only frustration and desperation.

Nutritional Healing in Polycystic Ovary Syndrome

The dietary advice for polycystic ovary syndrome is similar to that of insulin resistance, with the need to reduce carbohydrates more essential and challenging because of the complex hormone involvement. But it is just as important to be alert to the increasing dangers that external sources of synthetic hormones can add to the disruption of hormones in this condition. The good news is that polycystic ovary syndrome is manageable by diet, given a strict control over carbohydrates. Review the dietary advice for insulin resistance and make the following additions to help in the management of this condition.

Diet Management of Polycystic Ovary Syndrome
Reduce External Sources of Hormones
- Avoid meat, poultry, eggs and dairy raised on growth hormone
- Avoid using plastics, detergents, and household cleansers made from estrogen derivatives

Increase Fiber in the Diet
- Eat more fiber-rich fruits, vegetables, beans and legumes to increase transit time of the bowel and reduce hormones from being re-circulated in the large intestine
- Fiber helps to increase SHBG, reducing the amount of free

testosterone, which causes many of the male characteristics

Support the Liver to Improve Hormone Breakdown
- Increase foods that feed and nourish the liver, such as carrots, broccoli, Brussels sprouts, cabbage, cauliflower, beets, globe artichokes, lemons, watercress
- Decrease alcohol, caffeine and drugs

Supplements Helpful in Insulin Resistance
- Magnesium 400mg a day to reduce insulin resistance and help depression
- B-complex 50 to improve metabolism and liver function
- Vitamin C 500mg with bioflavonoid twice a day for the endocrine health
- Chromium 50mcg a day to support blood sugar levels
- Zinc 20mg a day to support the endocrine system and balance sugar
- Probiotics to help cleanse the gut and reduce candida

Herbal Healing in Polycystic Ovary Syndrome

The best advise to women with polycystic ovaries is to reduce stress and improve their blood sugar control, something herbal remedies do very well. With the ability to work through the nervous system, adrenal glands, liver and pancreas herbs offer women the capacity to positively affect the whole of the endocrine system and improve hormonal health. Good herbal remedies are beneficial in bringing balance to women with polycystic ovary syndrome, enabling them to manage not only their weight and appetite, but also their lives.

Aims of Herbal Healing in
Polycystic Ovary Syndrome

Balance Blood Sugar and Reduce Insulin Resistance
Sacred basil, basal, cinnamon, goats rue, gurmar, bilberry, globe artichoke, dandelion root, fringe tree, nettle leaf, alfalfa

Improve Liver and Pancreatic Function to Help Hormone Balance, Increase SHBG, and Balance Insulin Levels
Fringe tree, dandelion root, globe artichoke, milk thistle, barberry, Oregon grape root, blue flag, burdock

Provide Hormone-active Herbs where Appropriate
Chaste tree, peony, saw palmetto, sarsaparilla, black cohosh, hops, licorice, nettle root

Improve Adrenal Gland Function and Reduce Stress
Siberian ginseng, borage, schisandra, gotu kola, astragalus, ginseng, licorice, ashwaghanda, schisandra

Reduce Anxiety, Tension and Depression
Skullcap, betony, vervain, oats, valerian, St.John's wort, pulsatilla, damiana, passionflower, rose, chamomile, rosemary, lavender

Examples of Herbal Remedies for
Polycystic Ovary Syndrome

Polycystic Ovary Syndrome with Obesity and Insulin resistance

Alfalfa	20ml	balances blood sugar,
Basil	15ml	Improve metabolism
Gurmar	5ml	Reduces taste for sugar
Fringe tree	20ml	Improve liver and pancreas
Siberian ginseng	15ml	anti-stress, balance metabolism
Vervain	25ml	relaxing nerve tonic
	100ml	

Dose: 5ml (one teaspoon) three times a day

Polycystic Ovary Syndrome with Infertility

Nettle leaf	15ml	Balances blood sugar
Nettle root	15ml	Balance hormones
Gurmar	5ml	Reduces taste for sugar
Dandelion root	20ml	Balances blood sugar
Chaste tree	5ml	Balances hormones
Astragalus	15ml	anti-stress
Skullcap	25ml	Relaxing nerve tonic
	100ml	

Dose: 5ml (one teaspoon) three times a day

Polycystic Ovary Syndrome with Hirsutism

Goats rue	20ml	Balances blood sugar
Gurmar	5ml	Reduces taste for sugar
Globe artichoke	20ml	Improve liver and pancreas
Nettle root	20ml	Balances hormones
Licorice	15ml	Anti-stress
Damiana	20ml	Relaxing nerve tonic
	100ml	

Dose: 5ml (one teaspoon) three times a day

Polycystic Ovary Syndrome with Acne

Bilberry	20ml	Balances blood sugar, cleansing
Gurmar	5ml	Reduces taste for sugar
Blue flag	20ml	Cleanse through the liver
Sarsaparilla	15ml	Skin detoxifier
Gotu kola	20ml	Improve adrenal glands
Rose	20ml	Relaxing anti-depressant
	100ml	

Dose: 5ml (one teaspoon) three times a day

Healing Tools for Polycystic Ovary Syndrome

Aims of Healing
- Learning to forgive
- Self-acceptance
- Balancing masculine and feminine energies

Mediation for Polycystic Ovary Syndrome

With stress and negative emotions a part of the condition of polycystic ovary syndrome, meditation offers women an opening into their own healing. The time and stillness it brings can help them relax, bring more positive energy and draw them closer to understanding their true nature. This next meditation guides women gently into meditation, and is especially helpful for those with little experience of it.

Buy a nice large candle especially for this meditation. Find yourself a room where you can be alone and there is quiet. Light your candle, dim the lights of the room and sit comfortably in front of the candle. Take some deep breaths, releasing any tension and anxiety you may have and clearing away the negativity of the mind. Begin to focus on the flame in front of you. Make everything else leave your mind but the light of the candle. It can become a very relaxing and hypnotic experience. If other things come to your mind, return your focus to the candle. Sit like this for five minutes and when you feel you are ready, close your eyes and wander off into the empty space that has been created in your mind. In this space keep returning to the void in front of you and enjoy the peace and tranquility it brings. Remain in this place for another fifteen to twenty minutes and increase the time as you progress with it. When you feel ready, open your eyes and return your glaze to the candle, sitting quietly before returning to your everyday world.

Visualization for Polycystic Ovary Syndrome

When sitting comfortably in a relaxed room, close your eyes and envisage your blood stream full of two types of testosterone: one is testosterone which is attached to its carrier molecule and appears as a white ball; the other testosterone is traveling alone without the buffering affects of its carrier molecule and appears as a black ball. On looking at your blood stream you are able see the black testosterone balls overcrowding the white ones. Begin to see yourself removing the black testosterones with a tweezers and placing them in a glass of water. With each one you take out, you can see your blood stream looking less crowded and more free-flowing. See how it becomes more and more full of white balls. Continue until you have removed all the black ones and your blood stream contains only white ones. Take the glass of black testosterones and visualize yourself pouring them down the sink. After a deep breath open your eyes and enjoy the balance you feel.

This is a good exercise to do as often as possible to help balance testosterone levels. It can be done watching TV, sitting on a bus or working at your desk. With time, it can become a friendly game that is pleasant to do, sending all the right signals to your body.

Inner Child Visualization

Find a space where you can be alone and peaceful. Sit quietly with your eyes closed and take three deep breaths to release any tension and negative thoughts. You are about to take a tour of a beautiful mansion on a sunny warm day. Visualize a large Victorian mansion enclosed in a beautiful landscaped garden. You walk up to a white, wrought iron gate and peer through the spokes. You open the gate and walk along a driveway lined with flowering bushes of mock orange, roses and honeysuckles, the scent following you and making you feel relaxed and cheerful. You arrive at the front entrance of the house and it looks friendly, with white and pink geraniums lining the window boxes and a magnificent vine of wisteria covering the front entrance. It seems very welcoming and the housekeeper greets you at the front door with seven keys of all different colors. She invites you to come in and look at each of the rooms on the first floor. As you climb the oak paneled stairway you find seven different colored doors, each corresponding to the colors of the keys.

The first door you come to is the red room, which you open with your red key. As you enter you are surprised to find it is a nursery, all pink and lacey with a crib, the smell of baby power in the air and nursery rhymes playing gently in the background. It feels comforting in the room and there is a rocking chair by the window. You sit down for a moment and enjoy the sense of security you feel. The sun is pouring in on you as you rock and you are relaxed and safe. Think now about your own birth and the stories you were told surrounding it. Although it may be hard to remember, think about any traumas or sadness that occurred when you were this age. See if there is anyone in your life, around that time, that did not care for you the way they should have. If so, visualize yourself and the individual looking at each other and tell them how unsafe they made you feel by their actions. Then find it in yourself to forgive them. When you feel you have made amends, get up from the rocking chair and leave the room feeling secure in yourself.

You now make your way to the next door, the orange one, and place your orange key in. Here you find yourself in room full with toys, clowns and dolls. You are transformed back in time to your own days around the age of five to eight years old. You pick up a cuddly, stuffed animal or doll, like one you used to have and make your way to a soft, orange bean bag that you sink into feeling reassured and snug. Think back in your life to this age and see if there is anyone you need to forgive for hurting you or causing you harm. See them in front of you and tell them how they have hurt you. Then spend some time trying to forgive them. When you feel ready you can leave the orange room, feeling lighter in yourself and with the joy of a child.

In the hall, you make your way to the next room, the yellow room, which opens easily with the yellow key. It's a lively yellow room with drawings you made and pictures of things you used to like when you were about eight to twelve years old. There are bunk beds that you used to share with friends and your favorite cartoon is playing quietly on TV in the background. You like the positive energy of this room and you decide to sit on the fluffy yellow rug on the floor and think back to images of your life at this time. Think about this period in your life and if there were any people in it that would have caused you to feel bad about the person you were. If so, visualize them with you on the rug and tell them what you feel they have done to you. Now take some time to forgive them and, after that, get up and leave the room feeling more confident in yourself.

You find the next door, a green door, and open it. You feel a sense of warmth immediately as you enter the room, and your heart is transported back to a time in your life when you were about twelve to fifteen years of age. There is music from your teenage years playing in the background and on your bed is your open diary. The posters on the walls remind you of your first infatuations and dreams of love. You smile and are invited by the lovely pink bedspread to lie down and think about any heartbreaking experiences that may have occurred to you at that time of your life. See the people in front of you and tell them how much they broke your heart. Then find it in yourself to forgive them so you can move onto the next room. When you leave, you notice a gentle warmth coming from your heart that feels nice.

The next door is the blue one and, as you place the blue key in the door, it opens and you find yourself in a sky blue room full of the memorabilia of your youth. There may be pictures of old boyfriends and girlfriends on your dresser and you smile at the thoughts of these experimental years in your life, around the ages of fifteen to twenty years old. You sit in the window seat looking out into the distance and thinking about this time of your life. If someone stifled you and stopped you from being who you wanted to be, during these years, see them appear in the room and hear yourself express how they kept you back. Hear yourself say it in a strong, firm voice and then find it in yourself to forgive them. When you are ready, leave the room feeling proud of your power and strength.

You now find yourself in front of the indigo room and as you place the key into the lock, it opens and reveals a room that is the same as your bedroom now. There, in the corner, is your favorite chair. As you sink into the chair you are feeling happy with yourself and where you have come from. But if, within you, come feelings that stop you from feeling as well as you can, allow any personal conflicts that are presently niggling away, or relationships that are causing you pain, to surface in this room. See the people involved come to you in the room and explain to them just what they are doing to you. Now find the courage in yourself to forgive them. As they disappear from your view, you walk out the room feeling peaceful in yourself that you have transcended this uncomfortable situation.

Now you are at the end of the rooms, all that is left is the white key to the garden. In front of you is a large French door looking out into the garden. As you open the door you descend the stairway and walk out into the beautiful garden. The sun is shining, the birds are singing, the smell of sweet violets fills your nose with joy. There is a lightness in your step and you twirl around enjoying the beauty of nature. You feel free and happy and a part of this lovely energy.

You make your way down the path and out the gate, opening your eyes when you are ready.

Affirmations for Polycystic Ovary Syndrome
I love all that I am
I allow myself to be who I was born to be
I accept my feminine energies

Psychotherapy for Polycystic Ovary Syndrome
Learn how you may have reacted to the motives and energies of those who cared for you and how they may have affected your masculine and feminine energies.

Hands-On-Healing Exercise for Polycystic Ovary Syndrome
With an imbalance of masculine and feminine energies under-lying polycystic women, there is a need to restore balance and bring these energies together, working for the greater benefit of the women. In this exercise, the masculine energies of the sun are brought together with the feminine energies of the earth, equalizing, blending and vitalizing for the benefit of the woman.

This exercise can be done sitting, standing or lying down. Become conscious of your breathing and allow it to form a relaxed and regular pattern. Take a deep in-breath and as you begin to slowly breathe out, imagine you are pulling the golden energy of the sun into your head. As you slowly breathe out, feel it move down the left side of your body. Encourage your breath to last until you reach your feet.

With the next deep in-breath, imagine drawing the silver earth energies from the ground up from your feet. With your breath, follow this energy as it rises up your right side moving up your legs, hips, torso, shoulders, neck and head.

Now in the top of your head, see the two energies swirling and mixing and with the next out-breath, bring the two spiraling energies down through your left side and up the right side with the in-breath. Take some time coordinating the breathing and getting this into a nice relaxed flow. Try doing this for ten breaths.

Before you end, take one last deep breath and begin to see the gold and silver energy wrap around each other and form a helix, like in DNA. Watch as it enlarges and moves outward into the center of the body, filling the whole body with its pulsating energy, bringing balance and wholeness.

Endometriosis

Endometriosis is a condition where the tissue that lines the uterus, (the endometrium) wanders outside the boundaries of the womb. As it wanders it begins to implant itself and grow into a living glandular structure that responds to fluctuations in estrogen and progesterone, just like in the womb, causing contractions, pain and bleeding at these sites. This time the symptoms of menstruation are found, not only in the womb, but also in a number of other possible sites; some nearby, like the cervix, fallopian tubes, ovaries, bladder, bowels and vagina, and some less often found as far away as the lungs, kidneys and brain. The pain and discomfort women expect in normal menstruation becomes more intense and debilitating with endometriosis. With the growth of endometrium at these other sites, the associated symptoms can become more complicated and women may experience pain with defecation, urination and intercourse. As this abnormal tissue grows it can also develop into cysts, adhesions and infertility. The symptoms of endometriosis can look similar to other diseases, sometimes prolonging diagnosis and affecting treatment. It can spread, implant and regress, just the same as cancer does; its pain in the bowel is similar to that of irritable bowel syndrome; it can produce uncomfortability in the bladder that feels like cystitis; it can mimic the symptoms of appendicitis; it can be hard to distinguish from pelvic inflammatory disease and it can form cysts just like polycystic ovary syndrome. Endometriosis is a difficult hormonal condition for women to cope with, mostly for the severity of pain it can cause and the exhaustion it can bring, leaving women depressed, anxious and apathetic. Their wariness can often be seen in their eyes, showing just how much the condition has taken from them. From this, you can begin to understand why some women with endometriosis go to the extreme of having their womb removed to relieve their pain.

Physical

Endometriosis can be viewed as a hormonal condition of estrogen dominance, where estrogen loses its balance and begins to perform its activities in a more aggressive and damaging way. One of the functions of estrogen is to rebuild the womb lining with each new cycle. Women with endometriosis seem to have an exaggeration of this activity, caused by higher levels of estrogen circulating through their blood stream, mostly in an unbound state, without the protection of carriers and receptors to buffer its actions and be specific in targeting the correct tissues. In this highly active state, it can be transported through the blood and lymph to places outside the womb, where it implants and exerts its menstrual activities. The issue of most importance for endometriosis becomes finding the sources of excessive estrogen and reducing the imbalance at as many levels as possible. The first place to begin looking for the source of estrogen is at the women themselves to see if they are overweight and their fat cells are producing too much estrone, upsetting estrogen balance. The other place to look for answers is the liver, where estrogen balance is normally maintained by the degradation of estrogen into weaker forms, so it can be easily excreted through elimination channels. When liver function is reduced by an unhealthy diet, viruses or alcohol and drug abuse, there can be a reduction in estrogen degradation resulting in the re-circulated in its more active form. Liver health is further compromised by the increasing amount of exogenous estrogens found in the food chain, homes and in the environment which place a strain on its functions. Once passed through the liver, estrogens of all kinds pose another risk when they pass through the large intestine of women with candida. This is where the toxins produced by fungus are able to reconnect the bonds that have been previously broken in the liver, reactivating estrogen and resulting in its re-circulation and dominance, and enabling a condition like endometriosis to progress.

Emotional

The extreme symptoms of endometriosis should not occur in women that have an effective immune system that keeps unusual tissue from growing in unusual places. Nor should it come to women with healthy adrenal glands that stabilize hormone imbalances and keep pain from being so intense. What enables a condition like this to progress would have to be something that can cause these protective systems to fail. In following the stories of women with endometriosis, it becomes clear that many of them have histories of chronic stress in their lives. Stress hormones have the ability to, not only cause estrogen dominance, but also to reduce the immune capacity of women and exhaust the adrenal glands, producing conditions like endometriosis. When insecurity, instability and fear are part of young girls' early years, the adrenal glands mask their stresses by the producing stress hormones, hiding what they are really feeling inside, while also helping to detach them from their own issues and tissues. They grow into women who, in their 30's, get endometriosis at a time in their lives when a lot of their childhood dreams are becoming disillusions, their expectations are becoming disappointing and responsibilities are mounting. The stress of their early lives weakened their endocrine system and now, at an age when they are hormonally active, having babies and using contraceptives, they are diagnosed with endometriosis. Women who get endometriosis are women who have had to push themselves a little bit harder to get where they are because of their lives, and are usually driven to succeed, a way of concealing their inner self-doubt. Their serotonin levels tend to be low (possibility due to an underlying depression) and as the condition progresses, this becomes a factor in the intensity of pain they feel. With high cortisol levels, their progesterone levels can be reduced, increasing the stimulating power of estrogen to act on their tissues. With abnormal estrogen levels and high cortisol, the body is in a deteriorative state, with an immune system producing less immune compounds that normally prevent the endometrium tissue from growing and implanting in remote tissue. As this happens, there can also be an autoimmune response that is elicited when antibodies are produced against a tissue growing in the wrong place.

Spiritual

What brings the immune system of women to work against their own tissues is a deeply spiritual issue. Something within their lives has distanced them from their own energy and they have become disconnected from their soul. It is similar to what occurs in cancer, and in many ways endometriosis is very like cancer in the way it implants and spreads and in the quality of its pain. But what they also have in common is that they both arise from an exhaustion that occurs when unconditional love becomes conditional. Somewhere in their early lives, women with endometriosis may have struggled to be accepted and loved by one or another of their parents, causing their unconditional loving nature to become highly conditional to get their needs met. Some women may have been terribly let down by their mother, coming away feeling unsupported and vulnerable. Others may have found, early in their lives that their fathers' love was unattainable, and unconsciously made every effort to be more like him to gain his love, attention and approval. What both of these do is to turn young girls away from their open, encompassing and caring feminine energies, while giving power to their masculine energies, those that make them hardworking, self-contained, unemotional, and that hide their unconscious fear of their own feminine energies. In the womb there becomes a battle between these energies, with their aggressive masculine energy overpowering the womb and destroying its health and stability. Without the stability of unconditional love in their lives, these women are unable to love themselves enough to keep their tissues identifiable to their immune system, and through this, their tissues break down as if they do not belong to them.

Nutritional Healing for Endometriosis

In endometriosis, excessive estrogen levels can be seen as a toxicity to the body and every effort must be made to reduce incoming toxins and estrogens and to keep elimination organs performing as best as possible, both of which can be done through the diet. Many times the diet of women with endometriosis is not a healthy one, partly because of the conflicting energy running through them, and partly because of their detachment from their own needs. Nourishing themselves is a key to helping them find what feels right to them.

Diet Management of Endometriosis
Reduce Estrogens from the Diet and Increase their Elimination
- Increase fiber-rich fruits, vegetables, whole grains and bran to:
  - -improve bowel function
  - -limit the amount of estrogen able to be re-circulated
  - -balance gut organism
- Increase foods that support the breakdown of estrogen in the liver: carrots, beetroot, globe artichokes, broccoli, Brussels sprouts, cabbage, cauliflower, lemons, watercress, garlic, leeks and onions
- Eat only organic meats, poultry, eggs and dairy that have not been reared on growth hormones
- Reduce the use of plastics, detergents and household cleaners that are made from estrogen derivatives
- Decrease alcohol and caffeine as they both can reduces liver function, increasing estrogen levels

Foods to Increase Immune Health
- Increase sulfur-rich foods to improve immunity: garlic, onions, leeks

- Increase Vitamin C-rich fruits and vegetables: oranges, grape-fruits, tangerines, strawberries, raspberries, cranberries, guavas, kiwis, melons, cantaloupes pineapples, mangos apricots, tomatoes, asparagus, broccoli, cabbage, cauliflower, peppers, kale, parsley, potato, yams and all green leafy vegetables to:
    - -increase immune health
    - -improve adrenal gland health
    - -reduce abnormal cell growth
    - -improve healing and restoring of tissue
    - -reduce adhesions
- Avoid all sugars and sugar products, including white sugar, maple syrup, honey, molasses, dried fruits, cookies, candy, cakes, bakery products, processed cereals, fast foods, junk foods, colas, soft drinks and desserts which can disrupt estrogen levels through the excess production of insulin
- Eliminate refined carbohydrates: white bread, cake, cookies, bread crumbs, pasta and processed cereals
- Increase foods high in zinc for immune health: onions, garlic, parsley, eggs, sunflower seeds, pumpkin seeds, dairy, shellfish, herrings, beans, molasses, oysters, poultry, fish, seafood, lentils, almonds, peanuts, wheat germ, whole grains and dried fruits
- Eat foods high in omega 3 essential fatty acids to reduce inflammation: avocado, flax seeds, pumpkin seeds, salmon, tuna, herring, mackerel, sardines and anchovies
- Reduce red meats that are high in arachidonic acid and can make inflammation

Supplements Helpful in Endometriosis
- Magnesium 400mg to reduce muscular spasms
- B-complex 50 to help liver metabolism
- Vitamin C 500mg with bioflavonoid twice a day
- Zinc 20mg a day to support the immune system

- Vitamin E 400 IU a day
    -a natural antagonist to estrogen
    -reduce adhesions
    -inhibits the inflammatory process

Herbal Healing in Endometriosis

Conventional treatment of endometriosis usually entails putting more hormones into the body in the hope of balancing hormones levels. They do this by giving synthetic progesterone by injection, birth control pills or by a coil, to help balance out estrogen levels, or by drugs that inhibit pituitary hormones, preventing ovulation. Although these treatments may prevent the pain associated with endometriosis by stopping the cycle, they ignore the primary cause and do not help women feel any better in themselves. In fact, progesterone is a central nervous system inhibitor and can cause many women more depression, fatigue and exhaustion, especially at the doses given. Even laser treatments to reduce endometrial tissue in the womb are only temporary relief when nothing else has been done to change the progression of the condition itself. My personal experience even questions the use of estrogenic herbs, such as black cohosh, licorice, Chinese angelica and marigold, as they tend to create more complications only adding to the physical and emotional symptoms, particularly where candida coexists with endometriosis. Treating the women, is just as important as treating the hormones in this condition, and herbal remedies provide all that is needed to bring balance to both.

Aims of Herbal Treatment for Endometriosis
Reduce Pain
Jamaican dogwood, pulsatilla, valerian, passionflower, black haw, cramp bark, peony, motherwort, ginger, feverfew, raspberry, willow bark, meadowsweet, St John's wort, wild lettuce,

rosemary, chamomile

Balance Estrogen Levels through the Liver and Large Intestine
Dandelion root, turmeric, blue flag, globe artichoke, fringe tree, milk thistle, Oregon grape root, barberry, burdock, bayberry, agrimony, goldenseal, yarrow, feverfew

Balance Hormone Levels through the Pituitary Gland
Chaste tree, sarsaparilla

Cleanse, Tone and Heal the Endometrial Tissue
Ladies mantle, yarrow, blue flag, echinacea, goldenseal, Oregon grape root, barberry, bayberry, cleavers, poke root, echinacea, burdock, chamomile, raspberry, rose

Increase Circulation to Bring Cleansing and Healing
Ginger, blue flag, yarrow, prickly ash, gingko, hawthorn, cayenne pepper, basil, celery, echinacea

Improve Immune Health
Arbor vitae, echinacea, poke, cleavers, astragalus, baikal

Relax the Body and Mind and Reduce Depression
Skullcap, vervain, betony, St. John's wort, oats, rose, valerian, anemone, chamomile, Jamaican dogwood, lime blossoms, rosemary, wild lettuce, lavender

Improve Adrenal Gland Function, Reduce Cortisol Levels and Reduce Stress
Siberian ginseng, gotu kola, borage, ashwaghanda, licorice, astragalus, schisandra

Examples of Herbal Remedies for Endometriosis

Endometriosis with Pain

Pulsatilla	20ml	Pelvic pain relief
Raspberry	20ml	Reduce muscular pain
Ginger	5ml	Pelvic pain relief
Feverfew	5ml	Pain relief, liver balance
Jamaican dogwood	25ml	Pain relief, relaxing sedative
Ashwaghanda	<u>25ml</u>	Lower cortisol levels
	100ml	

Dose: 5ml (one teaspoon) three times a day throughout cycle. When in severe pain increase dose up to 10m per dose.

Endometriosis with Adhesions and Cysts

Black haw	25ml	Reduces muscular pain
Blue flag	20ml	Increases pelvic circulation
Arbor vitae	10ml	Reduces abnormal growths
Rose	20ml	Relaxing and comforting
Gotu kola	<u>25ml</u>	Reduces stress, adhesions
	100ml	

Dose: 5ml (one teaspoon) three times a day throughout cycle

Endometriosis with Infertility

Dandelion root	20ml	Balances hormones
Chaste tree	10ml	Balances hormones
Yarrow	20ml	Increases pelvic circulation
Oats	25ml	Nutritive nerve tonic
Astragalus	<u>25ml</u>	Reduces stress and adhesions
	100ml	

Dose: 5ml (one teaspoon) three times a day throughout cycle

Endometriosis with Candida

Oregon grape root	15ml	Cleanse gut, reduce candida
Echinacea	20ml	Reduces fungus and toxins
Baikal	20ml	Reduce stress of fungus toxins

Chamomile	20ml	Reduces irritations
Siberian ginseng	<u>25ml</u>	Anti-stress
	100ml	

Dose: 5ml (one teaspoon) three times a day throughout cycle

Endometriosis with Depression

Vervain	25ml	Relaxing nerve tonic
Ladies mantle	20ml	Tones reproductive tissue
Basil	15ml	Increases metabolism
St. John's wort	20ml	Anti-depressant
Borage	<u>20ml</u>	Reduces stress
	100ml	

Dose: 5ml (one teaspoon) three times a day throughout cycle

Healing Tools for Endometriosis

Aims of Healing in Endometriosis
- Becoming more aware of your own energy
- Learning to love yourself unconditionally
- Balancing masculine and feminine energies

Relaxing Meditation for Endometriosis

This exercise uses a relaxing visualization to move you into a meditative state more easily.

In a quiet room, sitting in a comfortable chair with your feet touching the floor, close your eyes and allow the body and mind to become restful. Image yourself sitting in the middle of a forest, with the wind blowing strongly through the trees. Take time to feel the strength of the wind blowing the limbs back and forth, hear the whistling sound of the wind and feel the power in the air. Then, slowly begin to feel the wind die down; see the movement in the trees and leaves begin to settle, the sounds become quiet and the force in the air gone, until you are sitting in the middle of a silent stillness.

Sit with this feeling for a few minutes until your body and mind quiet to the calm of the forest. Now allow yourself to drift into a thoughtless meditation. As time goes on, feel your body becoming weightless and your mind becoming limitless. If you begin to wander into thoughts again, bring your focus back to the stillness of the forest. Try to do for at least twenty to thirty minutes at a time. By doing this mediation often, you can become more attuned to your own energy and begin to experience your life more deeply. Your immune system will begin to work harder for you and in a more appropriate way.

Detachment Visualization for Endometriosis
Think about an important relationship in your life; one that has a certain draw to it; one that makes you feel anger, sadness or discomfort, even if the individuals are long gone from your life. It may be someone you have felt held you back, or maybe it is someone let you down. Bring this thought up when you are alone, and in a place you will not be disturbed.

Close your eyes and image a curtain is being drawn all around you, feeling a gentle darkness settling over you, which brings relaxation to the muscles and stillness to the mind. Sit for a moment enjoying the relaxing feeling. Begin to visualize yourself in the middle of a green grassy meadow, with wild flowers of all colors surrounding you. The sun is warm and shining brightly against a clear blue sky. Imagine yourself feeling content, peaceful and smiling. In the distance a person starts walking towards you. As they get closer, you begin to recognize them as the person in your life that stirs up uncomfortable feelings in you. With them face to face with you, allow any feelings to surface. Begin to see an attachment appearing between you both, running from your heart to theirs. The attachment can be made of whatever material seems fitting, whether it be a ribbon, rope or chain. Image yourself using an appropriate implement, like a scissor, pliers or chain saw and begin to undue the attachment between your hearts. Feel how hard or easy it is to accomplish. See it fall away from the both of you. Smile at each other before you see the individual turn and walk away.

Now again become aware of your surroundings, in the middle of the sunny meadow with the flowers all around you. You feel a sense of freedom come over you, a lightening of your mood and a sense of peace. Take in the beauty of your surroundings and feel the same sensations in yourself. Enjoy this feeling and when you are ready, open your eyes and return to the room.

Remember, do not worry about hurting the other person, negative attachments are not beneficial to anyone in the relationship, so you also do them a favor by letting go and freeing them to move on too.

Inner Child Work for Endometriosis

Sit in a comfortable chair with the sound of relaxing music in the background. Take a few deep breaths to allow yourself to release any tension and negative thoughts. See yourself arriving at the door of a house, it could be one you make up or one you know. The door is ajar and you walk in. Through the hall you see a doorway and peeking through you find a brightly lit kitchen with a child, head down, drawing at the table. As you walk into the room you recognize the kitchen as the one you were raised in. The table is in the same spot, the smell is the same and the child drawing at the table is you at a young age. Take time to allow any feelings to surface with this image.

You sit down next to your younger self but she seems to ignore you. She seems pensive and distant, a mood which you can remember. You ask her what she is doing but she does not answer. You ask her to draw how she is feeling for you and her reason for being so unhappy. Take time here and wait for her to draw her feelings. When ready, ask her to show you her drawing and see what has caused her so much unhappiness. After looking at her drawing you are able to comfort her and give her all the kindness, affection and attention she needs to make her happy. See her begin to smile as you show her you are able to provide all she needs. Tell her you will care for her now and watch over her, so she can remain happy and carefree. Ask her if she would like to come home with you. If she does, take her by the hand and lead her out of your old kitchen and through the door, bringing her into your present kitchen. See her happy and playful in her new home. If she isn't ready to leave, keep coming back to her when you can, making friends with her until she will leave with you. Enjoy the comfort that this relationship brings to you. When you are ready, open your eyes and come back into the room, bringing the child-like playfulness with you.

Affirmations for Endometriosis
  I am lovable
  I believe in the richness of my own energy
  I am proud of my feminine nature

Psychotherapy for Endometriosis
Work on the closest relationships in your life with a psychotherapist to understand what they taught you about love and how you thought you had to change to get it.

Hands-On-Healing Exercise for Endometriosis
With endometriosis, the sacral chakra and the heart chakra need balancing, bringing more wholeness to the women. Find a place where you can be alone. Sit or lie down in a comfortable position. Take a few good deep breaths, exhaling all your tension. Place your hands over your sacral chakra close to your ovaries, just below the bellybutton. Sit for three minutes, becoming familiar with the energy it contains. Then begin to visualize this space internally. See two different sized balls in this space. The ball on the left is red and so large it almost fills the whole of the left side. The ball on the right is yellow and very tiny, like a pea. Starting

with the left, red ball, imagine it reducing in size to fit comfortably in half of the space. Then go to the right side and imagine the yellow, pea-sized ball growing to fit in the space, becoming the same size as the red one. See the two balls containing the same amount of space and fitting nicely in the sacral area.

Now become aware if the energy has changed in the sacral area. Spend another three minutes with your hands over this area and feel any energy shifts, and enjoy the sense of stability and peace you may experience.

Take a few deep breaths, bringing the energy from your nose down into your sacral area and allowing the energy from these balls to mix and swirl around and become marbleized. In their blending you see them changing to an orange pulsing energy within the sacral chakra that keeps growing stronger and brighter. Enjoy the vibrancy of this orange energy for a moment. Remove your hands and image closing the sacral area up, as if it were a California poppy closing its petals at night, leaving only a hint of light coming through the top.

Now place your hands over your heart chakra, on the chest surrounding your lungs, heart and breast. Spend three minutes at this area feeling the energy which comes from it. Then begin to see this internal space filling with a soft and comforting green and pink mass of energy that brings feelings of comfort and love, filling your heart chakra and leaving you with a great sense of contentment. Stay with your hands over this area for another three minutes, feeling its energy.

When you are done, gently contain the heart chakra energy by imagining the chakra closing, like the leaves of a prayer plant at night, covering the chakra but leaving just a touch of light sneaking through. Enjoy the power and comfort of your energy.

Menopause

Before the advent of hormone replacement therapy (HRT), menopause was an inevitable change of life that women whispered about while getting through it. Today, instead of it being a developmental stage in women's lives, it has become a physical condition with a pharmaceutical drug that can stop it from occurring. Much of the information women are getting about menopause today is coming from marketing strategies to sell a product, rather than their own collective experiences and instincts. Unfortunately, such a good job has been done over the last thirty years to sell HRT, that women have begun to believe them and are becoming further removed from the signs and intuitions of their changing bodies. They come in for treatment before their menopause, fearful and ready to defend themselves from the drenching hot flushes, the sagging breasts, the wrinkling skin and loss of their sexuality that is being presented as inevitable to all women. Some have been fooled into thinking that if they take HRT they will go through menopause while on it, missing out on its symptoms and keeping aging at bay. However, by the number of women needing help after their experience with HRT, it only proves that they will go through menopause after stopping the drug, with symptoms sometimes more intense and dramatic than they would have been without HRT. Normal menopause enables the body to slowly get used to lessened estrogen levels, whereas HRT keeps estrogen levels falsely raised, so when women stop taking it there is a greater degree of adjustment to go through, with the possibility of more aggressive symptoms. There is no better time for women to get the facts right and understand the physical, emotional and spiritual realities of menopause, so they can make the best choices for themselves, and not have their lives defined by culture trends, but by a collective consciousness and intuitive knowledge.

Physical

Menopause is a time in women's lives when their bodies and minds are moving through a transitional phase and they may get hot flushes, night sweats, insomnia, forgetfulness and fatigue. It may be comforting to know that not everyone gets all these symptoms and that the amount of discomfort is very variable in women. More importantly, most women do not need help with their menopausal symptoms. Looking at menopause as a physiological process can help women reduce some of their fear. The process of menopause is a protective one, moving women away from their reproductive ability, saving their energy and resources as they age, for their own survival rather than for reproduction. Where their bodies have been dominated by the powerful ovarian estrogen, estridiol, in their reproducing years, in menopause they become dominated by the weaker estrogen, estrone, produced mostly in the adrenal glands and fat cells, but can also be produced in other organs such as the skin and kidneys. It is estrone which will carry them through the rest of their lives, producing similar affects and functions as estridiol has done previously but with less of the potency. What menopause really is then, is the period of time it takes for the body tissues to adjust to the change from estridiol to estrone. Since estrogen affects just about every tissue in the body, the symptoms that this conversion can cause are variable and individual in all women. The most commonly shared symptom of menopause is the infamous hot flush, which, in itself, causes many of the other uncomfortable symptoms, such as agitation, anxiety and insomnia. The hot flush originates at the temperature control center in the hypothalamus which maintains a constant and even body temperature through the body. Normally, when the body heats up, this center makes the necessary physiological changes to disperse the heat throughout the body and have it pass out through the pores of the skin as perspiration without much notice taken. But this regulatory activity is governed by the presence of ovarian estridiol, and in menopause when these levels are low, temperature regulation can become disrupted. So when the body heats up due to warm weather, overdressing, hot foods, warm drinks or stress, the hypothalamus is unable to make the necessary physiological changes as fast as it has done previously, resulting in women feeling a great rush of heat rising up the surface of their skin, bringing a dramatic, unnerving and distressful sensation. Just as it passes, they may also feel the cold, as the hypothalamus fails to create balance between these two extremes. The amount and duration of women's discomfort with the symptoms of menopause depends on how fast the hypothalamus learns to respond to adrenal gland estrone instead of ovarian estridiol.

Emotional

This very important issue makes adrenal gland health and function a big factor in determining how well women respond to menopausal changes, and how long and uncomfortable their transition period will be. If we acknowledge the adrenal glands' vital role in the stress response and their production of stress hormones, we can begin to appreciate how decisive emotional stress can be to the amount of estrone women make at menopause and their outcome of this transition. Many women come to menopause drained, exhausted and weary after living through bad relationships, having their children leave home, in the midst are caring for elderly parents, or burdened by financial and job restrictions, making them ill-prepared for this major event in their lives. They may be women that have relied on the energy and strength of their stress hormones to help them to cope through their lives, leaving them with adrenal glands that are as tired and low as they are. When called upon in menopause to produce enough estrone to get them through their menopausal adjustment, their adrenal glands could be unable to meet the demands of their changing bodies. The effort that has gone into making stress hormones can become exhausting to the other functions of the adrenal glands and limit their ability to make estrone when called upon. Without adrenal estrone coming up to buffer the impact of reduced estridiol from the ovaries, women can experience more severe menopausal symptoms and for much longer periods of time. This makes the outcome of menopause relate to, not only the past stress of women's lives, but also to how much stress they currently live under. With this in mind, it becomes unfair to say menopause causes women to become weepy, overly sensitive and hysterical when it may not be menopause, but more the inability of their adrenal glands to continue to cover up their emotions with stress hormones, as they have done for so many years, now that there is more demand on them. This is what makes menopause such a variable experience for women, being shaped and determined by their lives as much as their hormones.

Spiritual

In accepting that menopause is a developmental stage in women's lives, it means that they are not only passing through physical changes, but also changes which bring significant alterations to their awareness, changing the way they see, think and feel, and bringing new inspiration and creativity to their world. Without this change it would mean that women's female roles are limited to reproduction and there is no need for any further progression in their lives after that is done. Life is much more loving and giving than that, and women have much more to give once their childbearing years are ended. For this purpose they are presented in menopause with fluctuations in their hormones and neuro-transmitters, similar to those occurring at the luteal phase of their cycle, bringing a more inward focus that strengthens their attachment to their instincts and intuitions and which is their road to wisdom. But this time, estridiol is not there to cause inter-ference, as it can often do in the luteal phase, and instead of only lasting a week, as it does premenstrually, it is with them everyday.

This is what can bring such richness to the lives of menopausal women and cause them to thrive in their roles as teachers, leaders, advisors, managers and healers. Their ability to give stretches wider and deeper than themselves or their families now, and many begin to give back to their communities with a knowledge that is sharpened by intuition and broadened by age. Unfortunately, for this positive step to be achieved, women may experience, at the start of their menopause, the uncomfortable symptoms of confusion, inability to concentrate, clumsiness, forgetfulness and sluggishness as their bodies and minds try to get used to the changing array of hormones and neurotransmitters that refine their spiritual awareness. This short period of adjustment, often referred to as 'menopausal fog', is actually the beginning of menopausal women's spiritual growth that will progress with them through their postmenopausal days and which can lead to wisdom. It is sad to think that the two times in women's lives when they are closest to their spiritual nature, the luteal phase of the cycle and menopause, are the two most difficult experiences for them and the ones which cause them the most negative symptoms. It could be that, for some women, getting that close to their inner world is too painful an experience, and the thought of something like HRT, that could prevent them going there, seems a more comforting option. Although they may relieve their immediate uncomfortability with HRT, the potential to achieve the spiritual aspirations of menopause is lost, and some women become stranded in a stage of their life that has lost its purpose, leaving them confused, hurt and empty. Women should make sure they come to menopause free of the restraints of the past so it does not get in the way of them fully experiencing their spiritual evolution in menopause.

Nutrition Healing in Menopause

The adaptation of menopause generates some stress itself, as the body tries to find its balance again. It is a stress that can be lessened or prevented if women come to menopause well nourished and healthy, making their transition easier. When women ignore proper nutrition throughout their lives, eating processed and fast foods, eating foods with lots of sugar in them, drinking alcohol and not eating enough fruits and vegetables, their bodies will come to menopause ill-equipped and they could experience a more difficult time. It is unfortunate that young women often have a sense of invincibility about them, not feeling the repercussions of eating badly until many years later, and especially in menopause when health is so critical to outcome. But don't let that stop you, menopause can always be helped and supported with proper nutrition, not only to ease the symptoms of menopause, but also to encourage women's spiritual ascent with foods that enhance this and not hinder it.

Diet Management in Menopause

Increase Vitamin C- rich Foods to Improve the Workings of the Adrenal Glands and Reduce Menopausal Symptoms, Especially Hot Flushes

- Oranges, grapefruits, tangerines, strawberries, raspberries, cranberries, guavas, kiwis, melons, cantaloupes pineapples, mangos apricots, tomatoes, asparagus, broccoli, cabbage, cauliflower, peppers, kale, parsley, potatoes, yams and all green leafy vegetables

Eat Foods High in Plant Estrogens to Naturally Restore Estrogen Balance

- Apples, apricots figs, peaches, cherries, plums, watercress, fennel, parsley, alfalfa, garlic, potatoes, yams, pumpkin, corn, broccoli, seaweeds, carrots, olives, oats, brown rice, wheat, peas, sprouts, beans, soy products, nuts and seeds

Avoid Triggers of Hot Flushes

- Caffeine containing drinks, coffee, tea and energy drinks

- Hot drinks
- Alcohol
- Sugar and sugar containing foods
- Spicy and hot foods
- Big meals
- Emotional stress

Supplements Helpful in Menopause
- Magnesium 400mg a day to help mood
- B-complex 50 to improve metabolism and nerve and brain functions
- Vitamin C 500mg with bioflavonoid twice a day for the endocrine health
- Zinc 20mg a day to support the endocrine system

Herbal Healing in Menopause

The key in using herbs in menopause is that they are used to improve the overall well-being of women, making them stronger and more confident so they can handle this natural development and all it brings, and not just provide them with a natural hormone replacement. It is often the stresses and exhaustion in women's lives which actually create their inability to cope with the added physical and emotional changes that can occur in menopause, and not so much the menopause itself. With this in mind, herbal treatment should be geared at improving adrenal gland function to improve the way women respond to menopause and provide them with the comfort and support of nerve tonics and relaxants that will make them feel better in themselves. These are often enough to reduce the common menopausal symptoms such as hot flushes, insomnia and agitation, but for some of the more aggressive symptoms, estrogenic herbs are a great support. They are especially useful for women who are either trying to come off their HRT and for those who have previously been on HRT, when the hormonal implications becomes more complicated. In these cases, hormonally active herbs can support the restoration of hormone balance more quickly and without the uncomfortable symptoms. Herbs can be a great comfort to menopausal women when used appropriately and when they are encouraging the transition rather than restraining it.

Aims of Herbal Treatment in Menopause

Improve Adrenal Gland Function and Reduce Stress
Siberian ginseng, borage, schisandra, gotu kola, astragalus, ginseng, licorice, ashwaghanda

Help Reduce Anxiety, Tension, Depression and Improve Well-being
Skullcap, betony, vervain, oats, valerian, St.John's wort, pulsatilla, rose, chamomile, rosemary, motherwort, hawthorn, lavender

Balance Estrogen Levels with Plant Estrogens
Black cohosh, red clover, sage, licorice, hops, marigold, Chinese angelica, fennel, rosemary, yarrow

Support the Liver to Improve Hormone Balance
Fringe tree, dandelion root, globe artichoke, milk thistle, barberry, Oregon grape root, burdock, licorice, blue flag, yarrow, wild yam

Examples of Herbal Remedies for Menopause

Menopause with Hot Flushes and Night Sweats

Astragalus	20ml	Anti-stress, cooling temperature
Motherwort	25ml	Relaxing, reduces hot flushes
Rose	20ml	Cooling relaxant
Sage	20ml	Cooling plant estrogen
Dandelion root	<u>15ml</u>	Cooling liver herb
	100ml	

Dose: 5ml (one teaspoon) three times a day. Should take last dose at bedtime.

Menopause with Fatigue

Licorice	15ml	Improves stamina
Siberian ginseng	10ml	Anti-stress
Oats	20ml	Lifting nerve tonic, general tonic
St. John's wort	20ml	Improves mental well-being
Chinese angelica	15ml	Source of plant estrogen
Blue flag	20ml	Improves hormone balance
	100ml	

Dose: 5ml (one teaspoon) three times a day. Do not take last dose too close to bedtime.

Menopause with Loss of Concentration, Forgetfulness ,Clumsiness

Gotu kola	25ml	Promotes brain activity
Betony	25ml	Lifting nerve tonic
Rosemary	15ml	Improves brain activity
Black cohosh	20ml	Plant estrogen
Globe artichoke	15ml	Improve hormone balance
	100ml	

Dose: 5ml (one teaspoon) three times a day

Menopause with Emotional Issues (depression, anger, mood swings)

Ashwaghanda	25ml	Improve adrenal gland function
Skullcap	20ml	Relaxing nerve tonic
Vervain	20ml	Lifting nerve tonic
Hawthorn	20ml	Relaxing sedative
Yarrow	15ml	Relaxing plant estrogen
	100ml	

Dose: 5ml (one teaspoon) three times a day

Healing Tools for Menopause

Aims of Healing in Menopause
- Cleansing of old emotions to be ready for change
- Acceptance of the changes of menopause

- Developing spiritual awareness

Meditation for Menopause
Because menopause is a time women are more attuned to the natural world around them, this meditation takes them out into nature. Find a space in nature where you feel safe, comfortable and one which has always drawn you into a deeper place in yourself. It can be in the middle of a forest, amongst the mountains, sailing on the ocean, sitting by a waterfall, or just lying in the sun in your garden. What's important is to feel alone, peaceful and to be undisturbed. See yourself sitting down in this space, feeling warm and relaxed. Look around you and take in the good feelings of this place and feel yourself ease into it.

With your eyes open, begin to breathe in the freshness and vitality of this setting and breathe out the stale emotions and negative thoughts you carry deep within you. Allow time for them to loosen with each breath. Do this about five times, breathing as deeply as possible. Then relax and keep looking into the landscape. Breathe in the smells, hear the sounds, see the colors and feel the energies that are around you. Sit and just enjoy this space for anywhere from twenty minutes to an hour. A stillness will take hold of your body and mind during this time, and you will begin to feel your own energy melding with the energy around you. You may experience moments when you are unable to distinguish your own energy from that around you. Enjoy that place and stay with it for as long as possible, bringing with it an awareness of your own spiritual nature.

A Cleansing Visualization for Menopause
Find a space where you can be undisturbed. Light candles, oils and play soft relaxing music, or anything else that you feel would make this space special for you. Sit for a moment with eyes closed and accept this space and time, believing you deserve it. Take a deep in-breath, feeling your abdomen enlarging and your chest

rising, then slowly release your breath, imaging you are releasing all the tension and negativity in your body and mind. Repeat two more times. Sit for a moment and enjoy the calm and comfort you feel.

Imagine yourself on a walking journey in a land of gentle green hills. You stride along feeling how good it is to be in the outdoors with no sounds other than the soft wind blowing against your ears. You walk with ease, your body feels strong and you are happy. The sun brings a brightness to the landscape, making everything seem clearer and sharper. The sky is an intense blue with the slightest brushstrokes of white clouds moving in the horizon. You pass soft feathery grasses swaying in the breeze. You can smell the freshness of the earth and the air. You look around you and feel an intense sense of joy. Enjoy this feeling for a moment.

As you make your way over a small hill, you see before you many more hills in the distance, looking welcoming and friendly. Between you and them there lies a river valley that you must cross before you can get there. As you make your way down, you begin to hear the sound of water as it passes through the hollow of the hills. You can feel the energy picking up, as the sounds of the water become more noticeable. As you come to the bottom, before you is a shallow river that you must cross to continue the rest of your journey.

You sit against a boulder for a moment, enjoying the arousing energy filling the air, as water moves over and around rocks in its passage through the valley. As you breathe in this moist energy, you begin to feel a loosening up of your own old emotions and memories. Instead of feeling bad it feels good. You begin to feel ready to let things go. Take some time now and think about anything in your life you would like to get rid of, any uncomfortable feelings, bad habits, negative patterns, strange behavior, painful experiences and hurtful relationships. Allow each one to rise in your mind and visualize yourself forming it into a ball and flinging it into the running water and see it float away. Take as long as you need to feel fully free of your emotional burdens and send them down the river.

When you are ready, stand up and make your way to the edge of the river. You place your hands in the water and feel its warmth. As you begin to make your way across some stepping stones, you feel a thrill and lightness come over you. You begin to move more confidently, your steps becoming more like strides and your pride and energy soaring. The water seems so inviting and safe that, as you make your way into the middle of the river, you step off the rocks and stand with your feet touching the bottom of the riverbed, allowing water to pass over and under you, cleansing, purifying and liberating you. It feels exhilarating, as the water moves around your body and you spend some time delighting in this feeling.

When you are ready, you step back onto the stepping stones and make your way across the rest of the river. As you arrive at the bank, you are feeling invigorated, revitalized and positive. You sit down for a minute to dry off in the sun and look up before you and see the many hills that await you and feel enthusiasm and excitement for what lies ahead of you. Enjoy this sense of adventure and optimism for what lies ahead in your life. When you have spent some time with this exciting feeling, slowly make your way back into the room and open your eyes.

Inner Child/Aging Crone Work for Menopause
Go into a room where you will be undisturbed. Light a candle with a comforting smell, play some relaxing music and place a pretty and colorful shawl around you, a color or print that makes you feel happy. Sit in a comfortable seat or lie on a soft rug.

Close your eyes and take a few deep breaths to clear out negative residue and leave space for new possibilities. Envisage the room filling with a soft, dreamy lilac-colored cloud, with nothing and no one in it but you. Feel the gentle, relaxing and comforting feeling it brings to you as it fills the room. You sense a new energy moving within you, one that is positive, serene and contented. You look around this lovely space you have created and feel at peace in yourself.

In this space three figures begin to emerge from the lilac mist. The first one looks to be a little girl. As she becomes more distinct, you recognize this little girl as yourself. The other figure is coming through now and appears to be a young woman. Through the mist, you begin to see this figure emerging into the women you were in your 30's. The other figure appears to be a grey haired old woman and, as she rises out of the mist, it becomes evident that she is you in your eighties.

You ask these three to sit down with you, all four of you forming a circle. You place the lovely shawl in the middle of the circle. You notice that the little girl has a look on her face which seems sad and frightened. You tell her that she does not have to carry around the load of her troubles anymore as they are no longer a part of her life and you can support her with any issues she may have. You ask her to bring each trouble up one by one, and then place them on the lovely shawl in front of her. Give her some time now as she reveals her troubles to you. Soon she is finished and you notice she has a more child-like look on her face and she is smiling and lively. She gets up and dances innocently in the misty lilac background.

Now you look at the young woman you used to be. She looks tired, weary and worried. You tell her she does not have to bear all her problems alone and invite her to disclose her deepest sorrows and fears so you can support her through them. As she explains each one, she places them down   on the lovely shawl in front of you. Allow her the time to express herself fully and see yourself reassuring her. When she is done, you notice how relieved she looks, beaming with a new sense of calm enthusiasm. She too gets up now and dances around the lilac mist of the room with your inner child.

You are left facing the old crone you will become. She looks fearful, anxious and tired. You ask her to explain to you why she is feeling as she does in old age. Tell her to bring forward all the fears she has about ageing and any concerns that keep her from resting peacefully in her later years. Have her place them on the shawl as they come up. See how she slowly feels more calm and relaxed as she relates her last concern. Leave her with an assurance that you will always be looking after her so she has nothing to fear. See her smile with great warmth and satisfaction as she gets up and joins the others, dancing in the lilac mist.

You now begin to fold up the shawl, bringing each corner carefully together, ensuring that all the difficulties and sorrows of your life are secured within the shawl. Move to the open window in the room and shake out all your cares into the sky. See them float ways into the atmosphere. After you have watched them all disappear, give the shawl a good shake and place it back over your shoulders. Take a deep breath, taking in the contentment of the lilac mist and go join the others, dancing happily in the lilac background. Enjoy the feeling of wholeness and harmony that comes to you now. When ready, open your eyes and come back into your room.

Affirmations for Menopause
I trust in who I will become in menopause
I allow the changes of menopause to enrich my life

Psychotherapy for Menopause
Work on issues surrounding big disappointments in your life, which can keep you from moving gently into menopause and cause more fear of aging.

Hands-On-Healing Exercise for Menopause
In menopause it is the upper chakras, the brow and the crown, that will direct the development of, and provide access to,

your spirituality. Through them will come a clarity of insight, sharpening of intuition, broadening of perception and inspiration for creativity. Many times, the higher chakras become less accessible if the lower chakras are blocked by the residues of life experiences. This following exercise will help to clear the way, making the energy of the higher chakras more accessible.

Sitting down in a quiet room, focus on your breathing and begin to feel your body relax and your mind become settled. Feel your feet making contact with the floor and become aware of the narrow space that exists between your feet and the floor. Imagine that from that space comes up an energizing flow of red earth energy that begins to travel up your feet, through your ankles and up into your legs and thighs. Feel the tingling pulse that lingers as it moves. As it reaches your thighs allow it to pass into your root chakra at the pelvis. Feel this strong red energy move around this space, bringing a deep, grounding feeling before it bursts upwards. It arrives at the sacral charka in the pelvic cavity, its energy turning a fiery orange as you feel it sweep around the ovaries and womb, generating a sense of spontaneity. From here, it rushes forward into the solar plexus area in the abdomen, now flashing a yellow glow that you can feel moving within you and raising your confidence. A deep breath draws it into the heart and breast area, where it is transformed into a green energy that sweeps around the chest, bringing a warm comforting glow. The energy now surges upwards into the throat charka, causing the energy to turn blue and enclose the space with a strong feeling of your own individuality. With the momentum generated by this upward force, the energy enters the brow charka, at the forehead, where the blue color mixes with purple and forms a shade of indigo which fills the head with its pulsing energy. Feel its energy moving around the brain, energizing and opening. Spend a few minutes in the brow chakra, feeling the intensity of its color and following it as it drifts around the brain, bringing light, power and resourcefulness. When ready, allow for it be driven upwards into the crown chakra, at the top of the scalp. With the energy of the chakras being able to pass unhindered through the lower chakras, it has now picked up strength and power, developing into a mass of violet vibrating energy and is able to be met by the golden white light of universal energy just waiting at its doors, bearing the rewards of wisdom and insight. Spend some time with this energy and feel its enthusiasm, clarity and insight. When ready, open your eyes and come back into your space.

Index of Common and Latin Herb Names

Common Names	Latin Names
Agrimony	Agrimonia eupoatoria
Alfalfa	Medicago sativia
Aloe vera	Aloe barbadensis
Ashwaghanda	Withania somnifera
Astragalus	Astragalus membranaceus
Barberry	Berberis vulgaris
Baikal	Scutellaria bacalensis
Basil	Ocimum basilicum
Bayberry	Myrica cerifera
Betony	Stachys betonica
Bilberry	Vaccinium myrtillus
Black cohosh	Cimicifuga racemosa
Black haw	Viburnum prunifolium
Blue flag iris	Iris versicolor
Borage	Borago officinalis
Burdock root	Atricum lappa
Celery	Apium graveolens
Chamomile	Matricaria recutita
Chaste tree	Vitex agnus castus
Chinese angelica	Angelica sinensis
Cinnamon	Cinnamomun cassia
Cleavers	Galium aparine
Cayenne	Capsicum minimum
Damiana	Turnera diffusa
Dandelion root	Taraxacum officinalis radix
Dandelion leaf	Taraxacum officinalis folia
Echinacea	Echinacea purpurea
Fennel	Foeniculum vulgaris
Feverfew	Tanacetum parthenium
Fringe Tree	Chionanthus virginicus

Garlic	Allium sativum
Galangal	Alpinia officinarum
Ginger	Zingiber officinalis
Gingko	Gingko biloba
Globe artichoke	Cynara scolymus
Goats Rue	Galega officinalis
Goldenseal	Hydrastis canadensis
Gotu kola	Hydrocotyle asiatica
Ground Ivy	Glechoma hederacea
Gurmar	Gymnema sylvestre
Hawthorn	Cratagus oxyacantha
Hops	Humulus lupulus
Ladies mantle	Alchemilla vulgaris
Lapacho Tree	Tabebuia impeteginosa
Lavender	Lavendula officinalis
Licorice	Glycyrrhiza glabra
Linden blossoms	Tilia europa
Marigold	Calendula officinalis
Marshmallow	Althea officinalis radix
Milk Thistle	Silybum marianum
Meadowsweet	Filapendula ulmaria
Motherwort	Leonarus cardiaca
Nettle leaf	Urtica dioica folia
Nettle root	Urtica dioica radix
Oats	Avena sativa
Oregano	Oreganum vulgaris
Oregon grape root	Berberis aquifolium
Passion flower	Passiflora incarnata
Peony	Peonia laciflora
Ribwort plantain	Plantago lancelata
Poke root	Phytolacca Americana radix
Pulsatilla	Anemone pulsatilla
Prickly Ash	Zanthoxylum clavaherculis
Raspberry leaf	Rubus idaeus

Red Clover	Trifolium pratense
Rose	Rosa damascena
Rosemary	Rosmarius officinalis
Sage	Salvia officinalis
Sacred Basil	Ocimum sanctum
Saint John's wort	Hypericum perforatum
Sarsaparilla	Smilax officinalis
Saw Palmetto	Serenoa serrulata
Schisandra	Schisandra sinensis
Siberian Ginseng	Eleutherococcus senticosis
Skullcap	Scutellaria lateriflora
Slippery Elm	Ulmus fulva
Sweet Wormwood	Artemisia annua
Thuja arbor vitae	Thuja occidentalis
Thyme thymus	Thymus vulgaris
Tumeric	Curcuma longa
Valerian	Valeriana officinalis
Vervain	Verbena officinalis
Wild Yam	Dioscorea villosa
Yarrow	Achilla millifolium

Useful Contacts

UK

National Institute of Medical Herbalists (NIMH)
Elm House
54 St Mary Arches Street
Exeter
Devon
EX4 3BA

Phone   01392-426022
Email   nimh@ukexeter.freeserve.co.uk
Web   www.nimh.org.uk

National Federation of Spiritual Healers (NFSH)
Old Manor Farm Studio
Sunbury-on-Thames
Middlesex
TW16 6RG

Phone   01932-783164
Email   office@nfsh.org.uk
Web   www.nfsh.org.uk

USA

American Herbalists Guild
141 Nob Hill Road
Cheshire, CT 06410

Phone   203 272-6731
Email   ahgoffice@earthlink.net
Web   www.americanherbalistguild.com

Healing in America (NFSH in America)

PO Box 432

Ojai, California 93024

Phone   805 640 0211

Email   info@healinginamerica.com

Web   www.healinginamerica.com

Australia

National Herbalists Association of Australia

PO Box 45

Concord West

NSW 2138

Phone   02 8765 0071

Email   nhaa@nhaa.org.au

Web   www.nhaa.org.au

New Zealand

National Federation of Spiritual Healers of New Zealand (NFSH)

PO Box 764

Thames

New Zealand

Phone   64 7868 5204

Email   bob.jan@xtra.co.nz

Web   www.nfsh.org.nz

Sources Consulted

Chapter 1

Asso, Doreen. *The Real Menstrual Cycle.* John Wiley & Sons Ltd, Chichester UK, 1983.

Barnard ND, et al. *Diet and Sex-Hormone Binding Globulin, Dysmenorrhea, and Premenstrual Symptoms.* Obstetrics and Gynaecology 2000 Feb; 95 (2): 245-250.

Barnes, Broada O., and Galton, Lawrence. *Hypothyroidism: The Unsuspected Illness.* Harper & Row Publishers, New York, 1976.

Berne, Robert, M. and Levy, Matthew N. *Principles of Physiology.* Mosby, London, 1996.

Graham, Effie, Stewart, Martha, and Ward, Penelope. *Seasonal Cyclicity: Effect of Daylight/Darkness on the Menstrual Cycle.* Menstrual Health in Women's Lives. University of Illinois, 1992, pp. 254-260.

Griffin, James E., and Ojeda, Sergio R. *Textbook of Endocrine Physiology.* Oxford University Press, 1996.

Kamilaris, TC., et al., *Effects of Altered Thyroid Hormone Levels on Hypothalamic-Pituitary-Adrenal Function.* Department of Medicine, Vanderbilt University School of Medicine, Nashville, Tennessee 37232. 1987, Journal of Clinical Endocrinology and Metabolism Vol 65: 994-999.

Lee, John, MD. *Natural Progesterone: the multiple roles of a remarkable hormone.* Jon Carpenter; 2Rev Ed 15 July 1999.

Llewellyn-Jones, Derek. *Fundamentals of Obstertrics and Gynaecology.* 6th Ed, Mosby, 1994.

Patrone, C., et al. A. *Cross-Coupling Between Insulin & Estrogen Receptor in Human Neuroblastoma Cells.* Milano Molecular Pharmacology Lab, Institute of Pharmacological Sciences, University of Milan, Italy. Molecular Endocrinology 1996, May, 10 (5): 499-507.

Sandyk, R. *The Pineal Gland and the Menstrual Cycle.* Department of

Psychiatry, Albert Einstein College of Medicine Montefiore Medical Center, Bronx, New York 100461. International Journal of Neuroscience 1992 Apr, 63 (3-4): 197-204.

Siberstein, SD, Merriam GR. *Physiology of the Menstrual Cycle.* Jefferson Headache Center, at Thomas Jefferson University Hospital, Philadelphia, PA 19107.Cephalalgia 2000 Apr; 20 (3): 148-154.

Tortora, Gerard J. and Reynolds Grabowski, Sandra. *Principles of Anatomy and Physiology.* HarperCollins College Publishers. 7th Ed. 1993.

Weideger, Paula. *Menstruation & Menopause: The Physiology and Psychology, the Myth and the Reality.* Alfred A. Knopf Publishers, New York, 1976.

Chapter 2

Curry, A.S., Hewitt, J. V. *Biochemistry of Women: Clinical Concepts.* CRC Press, Cleveland Ohio, 1974.

Dye, L., Blundell, JE. *Menstrual Cycle and Appetite Control: Implications for Weight Regulation.* Human Reproduction 1997, Jun:12(6):1142-51.

Gannon, Linda R. *Menstrual Disorders and Menopause: Biological, Psychological and Cultural Research.* Praeger Publishers, New York, 1985.

Golub, Sharon. *Premenstrual Changes in Mood, Personality, and Cognitive Function.* Menstrual Health in Women's Lives. University of Illinois, 1992, 237-245.

Graham, Effie A. *Cognition as Related to Menstrual Cycle Phase and Estrogen Level.* The Menstrual Cycle. Vol 1: A Synthesis of Interdisciplinary Research. New York, Springer, 1980.

Mastorakos G, Zapanti E. *The Hypothalamic-Pituitary-Adrenal Axis in the Neuroendocrine Regulation of Food Intake and Obesity: the role of corticotropin releasing hormone.* Nutritional Neuroscience 2004, Oct-Dec;7(5-6):271-80.

O Caticha, WD. et.al. *Estradiol Stimulates Cortisol Production by*

Adrenal Cells in Estrogen-Dependent Primary Adrenocortical NodularDysplasia. Department of Internal Medicine, University of Utah School of Medicine, Salt Lake City 84132. Journal of Clinical Endocrinology & Metabolism, Vol 77, 494-497, 1993.

Parlee Brown, Mary. *Positive Changes in Moods and Activation Levels during the Menstrual Cycle in Experimentally Naïve Subjects. Menstrual Health in Women's Lives.* Psychology of Women Quarterly, 1982, 7 (2), 119-131.

Paxton, Mary Jean Wallace. *The Female Body in Control: How the Control Mechanisms in A Woman's Physiology Make Her Special.* Prentice Hall Trade Publishers, New Jersey 1981.

Selye, H. *The Stress of Life.* McGraw Hill, New York, 1978.

Witherspoon, James D. *Human Physiology.* Harper & Row Publishers, New York, 1984.

Wurtman, J. J., *Depression and Weight Gain: The Serotonin Connection.* Massachusetts Institute of Technology, Cambridge 02139. Journal of Affective Disorders 1993, Oct-Nov;29(2-3):183-92.

Chapter 3

Bolen, Shinoda Jean, *Goddesses in Everywoman: A New Psychology of Women.* Harper Colophon Books, New York, 1984.

Colegrave, Suki. *The Spirit of the Valley: A Jungian and Taoist Exploration of the Masculine and Feminine in Human Consciousness.* Virago Press Ltd, London, 1979.

Crook, William, G. *The Yeast Connection.* Vintage Books USA 1986.

de Castillego Claremont, Irene. *Knowing Woman: A Feminine Psychology.* Shambhala, Boston, 1997.

George, Demetra. Mysteries *of the Dark Moon: The Healing Power of the Dark Goddess.* Harper, San Francisco, 1992.

Gray, Miranda. Red *Moon: Understanding and Using the Gifts of the Menstrual Cycle.* Vega Books, USA 2002 and Element Books UK 1994.

Harding, Esther M. *Women's Mysteries: A Psychological*

Interpretation of the Feminine Principle as Portrayed in Myth, Story and Dreams. Shambhala, Boston, 2001.

Myss, Caroline. *Anatomy of the Spirit: The Seven Stages of Power and Healing.* Bantan Books, New York, 1996.

Owen, Lara. *Her Blood Is Gold: Celebrating the Power of Menstruation.* Harper, San Francisco, 1993.

Shuttle, Penelope and Redgrove, Peter. *The Wise Wound: Menstruation and Everywomen.* Marion Boyars Publishers, USA, 2005.

Shuttle, Penelope and Redgrove, Peter. *Alchemy for Women.* Ramboro Books, USA 1997. and Random House, London, 1994.

White, Ruth. *Working With Your Chakras,* Piatkus Publishers, 1994.

Chapter 4 and Section II, The Conditions

Angelo, Jack. *Your Healing Power: A Comprehensive Guide to Channelling Your Healing Energies.* Judy Piatkus Publishers, London, 1994.

Arvigo, Rosita. Rainforest Home Remedies: *The Maya Way to Heal Your Body and Replenish Your Soul.* Harper, San Francisco, 2001.

Bartram, *Thomas. Bartram's Encyclopedia of Herbal Medicine.* Constable & Robinson Ltd. London,1995.

Bradshaw, John. *Homecoming: Reclaiming & Healing Your Inner Child.* Bantam Books, New York, 1992.

Brennan, Barbara Ann. *Hands of Light: A Guide to Healing Through the Human Energy Field.* Bantam Books. New York, 1988.

Dethlefsin, Thorwald and Dahlke, Rudiger. The Healing Power of Illness. Element Books, 1997 UK.

Elias, Jason and Ketcham, Katherine. *In the House of the Moon: Reclaiming the Feminine Spirit of Healing.* Time Warner Books, New York, 1995. and Hodder & Stoughton, UK 1996.

Gladstar, Rosemary. *Herbal Healing for Women.* A Fireside Book, Simon & Schuster, New York, 1993.

Green, Julia, et al. *Treatment of Menopausal Symptoms by Qualified*

Herbal Practitioners: A Prospective, Randomized Control Trial. Family Practice, 2007; 1-7.

Greer, Germaine. *The Change: Women, Ageing and the Menopause.* Penguin, London, 1992.

Hall, Judy. *The Wise Woman: A Natural Approach to the Menopause.* Element Books, UK, 1997.

Hay, Louise L. *You Can Heal Your Life. Hay House Publishers,* California USA 1987 and Eden Grove Editions, UK 1988.

Loch EG, Selle H, Boblitz, N. *Treatment of Premenstrual Syndrome with a Phytopharmaceutical Formulation Containing Vitex agnus castus.* Journal of Womens Health, Gender Based Medicine 2000 Apr; 9

Murray, Michael, and Pizzorno, Joseph. *Encyclopedia of Natural Medicine,* 2nd ed., Pima Publishing, USA 1998.

Northrup, Christiane, MD., *Women's Bodies, Women's Wisdom: Creating Physical and Emotional Health and Healing.* Bantam Books, New York, 2002 and Piatkus, London, 1998.

Ojeda, Linda. *Menopause Without Medicine.* HarperCollins Publishers, London, 1990.

Ojeda, Linda. *Exclusively Female: A Nutritional* Guide *for Better Menstrual Health,* Hunter House, USA, 1983.

Page, Christine, R. *Frontiers of Health: From Healing to Wholeness.* Random House, New York, 2005. and C.W. Daniels Co, London 2000.

Pitchford, Paul. *Healing with Whole Foods.* North Atlantic Books, Berkeley, California, 2002.

Ritchie, Margaret, et al. *A Newly Constructed and Validated Isolflavone Database for the Assessement of Total Genistein and Daidzein Intake.* British Journal of Nutrition 95 (1): 204-213, Jan 2006.

Rogers, Carol. *The Women's Guide to Herbal Medicine.* Hamish Hamilton, London, 1997.

Saifer, Phyllis, Zellerbach, Meria. Detox: *A Successful and*

Supportive Program for Freeing Your body from the Physical and Psychological Effects of Chemical Pollutants. Ballantine Books, 1986.

Stevinson C, Ernst E. A Pilot Study of Hypericum perforatum for the Treatment of Premenstrual Syndrome. International Journal of Obstetrics and Gynaecology, 2000 Jul; 107 (7): 870-6.

Walker, Barbara, G. *The Crone: Woman of Age, Wisdom and Power.* Harper, San Francisco, 1988.

Index

Graves Disease, 67
Hashimoto's, 67
Lupus, 67
response, 110
Autonomic Nervous System
(ANS), 12, 24, 33-34, 37, 62,
78, 81
Awareness, 39, 56-57, 59, 61
confused, 71
heightened, 95
menopause, 180
spiritual 91
Back, 105
Baikal, (Chinese skullcap), 114,
129, 170
Baldness, 150
Basil, 114, 116, 129, 155
sacred, 90, 114, 116, 129,
155
Barberry, 115, 129, 170, 184,
185
Bayberry, 170
Behavior, 55
attention seeking, 68
negative, 30-31
Belly, pot, 122, 150
Betony, 90, 115, 129, 130, 140,
155, 170, 185
Betrayal, 40
Betrayed, 103
Bilberry, 115, 129, 130, 155
Biological processes, 15
Birth, 20, 41, 48, 55, 59, 63
Birth control pills, 14, 59, 74,

108, 111, 136, 169
Black cohosh, 155, 184, 185
Black haw, 169
Bladder, 88
Bleeding,
heavy, 14, 21, 72, 86, 88, 108
endometrial, 163
Blood, 17, 103
flow, 23
pressure, 14
supply, 35
vessels, 14
Blood Sugar, 2, 14, 20, 21, 36,
45-46, 69, 79, 126,
128, 166
balanced, 83
erratic, 152
herbs, 88
insulin resistance, 124, 126
irregularity, 45
premenstrual syndrome,
136
polycystic ovary syndrome,
151-152, 154-155
Blue flag iris, 129, 155, 156,
170, 185
Bone, 17, 103
Borage, 115, 141, 155, 170, 184,
Boundaries,
personal, 117, 121
Bowel, 74
endometriosis, 163
regularity, 17
Brain, 10-12, 17, 33-34, 37, 40,

Diarrhea, 108-109
Disappointment, 59, 103
DNA, 4, 162
Dopamine, 38, 39, 43, 47, 48,
    49, 57-58
    premenstrual syndrome,
    136
Drinking, 31, 80
Drugs, 31, 80, 153
    abuse, 164
    anti-inflammatory, 109
    pharmaceutical, 109, 177
    prescription, 105
Dysfunctional, families, 73
Dyslexia, 43, 105

Ears, 67
Eating,
    comfort, 45
    disorders, 45, 67, 70, 105
    emotions of, 81-84
Echinacea, 115, 170
Eczema, 19, 36
Edgy, 48, 50, 58
Eggs, unfertilized, 22-23
Ego, 61, 68, 96
Emotional,
    blocks, 37, 94
    disturbances, 38
    health, 83
    impulses, 40
    instability, 45-46, 110, 125
    issues, 185
    needs, 45

stability, 37, 61, 83, 108, 110
stress, 37, 41, 42
trauma, 32-33, 103
triggers, 33, 98, 99, 101
Emotional Center of the brain,
    33, 43, 62, 63
Emotions, 12, 30-32, 37, 53
    herbal medicine, 88-89
    negative, 31, 33, 38
    premenstrual syndrome,
    136-137
    repressed, 101, 136
Endocrine System, 10-12, 19,
    24, 30, 33-34, 60-62, 78, 100,
    115, 128, 137, 154, 163, 165
    food, 83-86
    restore, 115
    premenstrual syndrome,
    137
Endometrium, 110, 163, 170
Endometriosis, 2, 18, 20, 26, 33,
    43, 69, 72, 105,
    151, **163-176**
    adhesions, 163
    adrenal exhaustion, 165
    cancer, 163
    candida, 108, 110, 171
    cortisol, 165
    emotional aspects of, 165-
    166
    infertility, 163
    Jamacian dogweed, 88
    liver, the, 164
    pain, 163

Vitamin A, 82

Vitamin, B complex, 82, 83, 113, 128, 139, 154, 158, 183

Vitamin B_6 29

Vitamin C, 83, 128, 139, 154, 168

adrenal glands, 83, 182

foods, 182

Vitamin E, 83, 169

Vocal expression, 61

Voice, 17

Vulnerable, 16, 31, 35, 44, 166

Vulnerabilities, 84, 90, 94, 120

Waist line, 122

Water retention, 14, 18, 24, 26, 39

Weight, 29, 43, 122

gain, 14, 15, 149

obsession, 45

over, 122, 164

premenstrual syndrome, 136

Well-being, 17, 31, 32, 38, 40, 43, 57, 62, 63, 80, 87, 102, 183

Western culture, 91

White blood cells (WBC), 19, 43

White coating, candida, 112

Wild lettuce, 169

Wild yam, 184

Will to Live, 44, 65-66

Willow bark, 169

Wind, 109

Wisdom, 52, 53, 54, 61, 64

feminine, 53

food, 84

menopause, 180

Womanhood, 30, 55, 56, 103

Women's ,

chemistry, 34, 40, 55, 60, 74

hormones, 11, 12, 34, 65, 86

stories, 3, 30, 44, 45, 68, 69, 100, 102, 124, 159, 165

spirit, 74, 87

spiritual nature, 60

Womb, 20, 73, 163, 169

lining, 21, 23, 57, 83

Worthiness, 68

Wormwood, sweet, 114, 115

Wounded spirit, 50, 66, 99

Wounds, 52, 61, 71, 76-77, 112, 152

ovaries, 71

Yarrow, 170, 184, 185

Yeast, 109, 113

Yeilding, 57

Yin and Yang, 64

Zinc, 82, 128, 154, 168, 183

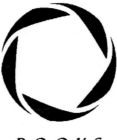

BOOKS

O is a symbol of the world, of oneness and unity. In different cultures it also means the "eye," symbolizing knowledge and insight. We aim to publish books that are accessible, constructive and that challenge accepted opinion, both that of academia and the "moral majority."

Our books are available in all good English language bookstores worldwide. If you don't see the book on the shelves ask the bookstore to order it for you, quoting the ISBN number and title. Alternatively you can order online (all major online retail sites carry our titles) or contact the distributor in the relevant country, listed on the copyright page.

See our website **www.o-books.net** for a full list of over 500 titles, growing by 100 a year.

And tune in to myspiritradio.com for our book review radio show, hosted by June-Elleni Laine, where you can listen to the authors discussing their books.

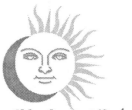

MySpiritRadio
31901050570714